PROFILES OF THE NUTRIENTS

1. CARBOHYDRATE, LIPID AND PROTEIN

PROFILES OF THE NUTRIENTS

1. Carbohydrate, Lipid and Protein

RICHARD RYDON

Non-fiction

First Paperback Edition: November 2016

ISBN: 978-1-326-80476-3

Cover image – ID 7499030 – tonobalaguer/123RF.com

Contents

Preface

1. The Meaning of Essential
2. Introduction to the Nutrients
3. Body Composition and the Nutrients
4. Water
5. Oxygen
6. Energy Requirement
7. Energy Metabolism
8. Energy and a Balanced Diet
9. Digestion
10. Food
11. Carbohydrates (and Organic Acids)
12. Dietary Fibre
13. Lipids
14. Fatty Acids (and Cholesterol)
15. Essential Fatty Acids: Linoleic Acid and α–Linolenic Acid
16. Proteins (and Nucleic Acids)
17. Amino Acids
18. Leucine
19. Lysine
20. Phenylalanine and Tyrosine
21. Valine
22. Threonine
23. Isoleucine
24. Methionine and Cysteine
25. Histidine
26. Tryptophan
27. Arginine

28. Protein Quality

A1. Solid and Liquid Portions Commonly Used in Cooking
and Dietetics

A2. Some Individual Fatty Acids

A3. Common Toxicity and Deficiency Symptoms
of Macronutrients

Bibliography

About the Author

Preface

This series of three books includes an account of the nutrients known to be essential for human life. Appropriately, the text is called PROFILES OF THE NUTRIENTS. The series covers some fifty different nutrients. It is intended primarily as an outline for those who seek an introduction to the nutrients presented in a direct way.

The classical definition of a nutrient is an essential substance in food that provides structural or functional components or energy to the body. The ability to provide energy requires one other essential substance that does not come from food, namely oxygen gas.

There are no value judgements on the special merits of selected nutrients. All are equally essential for human life. Each nutrient is identified in the text by:

- A Chapter of its own
- Common name and alternative names
- Some key historical dates (e.g. for the discovery of the vitamins)
- The Nature of each nutrient
- Biological functions
- Daily requirement and food sources
- Toxicity symptoms
- Deficiency symptoms

Book 1 considers carbohydrate, lipid and protein, book 2 considers minerals and trace elements and book 3 considers vitamins. Overall, the series presents a concise outline of each of the essential nutrients.

1

The Meaning of Essential

It is appropriate at the start to consider the meaning of the word *essential* as it applies to various nutrients. Several different shades of meaning of the term have been used. Five grades of essentiality can be distinguished ranging from absolutely essential to nonessential.

Absolutely Essential

Most of the nutrients are absolutely essential, that is to say they are indispensable in the diet, and are required in their own right. Many essential vitamins and minerals may be stored in the body. Consequently, the lack of supply of such nutrients in the diet may be tolerated, for temporary periods of varying duration, until the supplies are used up. Such a situation does not diminish the absolute essentiality of a nutrient only its temporary dietary requirement.

Indirectly Essential

Some nutrients, such as most of the carbohydrate, lipid and protein, are only indirectly essential for the purpose of providing sufficient energy. In many respects most of the lipid is only indirectly essential also, to ensure an adequate supply of essential fatty acids and fat-soluble vitamins, and to ensure their proper absorption.

Conditionally Essential

A number of nutrients may be termed conditionally essential, either because they are only required during certain periods of growth, such as the amino acids histidine and arginine, or because they can be synthesised in the body, like vitamin D in the presence of sunlight, or by the bacteria in the intestine, such as biotin and vitamin K. Circumstances may arise when nutrients must be supplied in the diet to fully meet nutritional needs, in which case they may be referred to as conditionally essential nutrients. But, unlike absolutely essential nutrients, they may not be required to the same degree throughout life. Conditional nutrients are those where the rate of synthesis in the body does not always fully match the requirement. Under a given set of circumstances, the nutrient must therefore be supplied in the diet, but under other circumstances it need not be.

Possibly Essential

Again, a small number of nutrients, notably certain trace elements, seem to be essential for several species and may also be essential for human metabolism. Such nutrients may be termed possibly essential. Many of these, even if they are essential, are required in such minute amounts that deficiencies in humans have not (yet) been established.

Nonessential

Finally, there are a large number of substances which are not essential in the human. The non-vitamins fall into this group. Many of these substances, while dispensable as nutrients, may have certain therapeutic effects if taken as supplements.

All the nutrients termed non-vitamins generally fall into the nonessential category. There is however a remote possibility that under certain circumstances some of these may verge on becoming conditionally essential. But, taking the strict view that nutrients should be classified on the basis of normal healthy requirements rather than requirements during exceptional illnesses or genetic disorders, it is usual to generally consider them as nonessential.

2

Introduction to the Nutrients

A nutrient is any substance needed by a living organism to maintain life. Every nutrient has special or unique properties essential for life. These properties are in some way related to the physical or more often the chemical nature of the nutrient.

Each form of life requires its own set of nutrients. This book, however, concentrates mainly on the requirements of the human body. It is intended as a concise yet comprehensive introduction to the nutrients.

In general language, the term nutrient is often used to refer to any and all components of food and even to whole foods. To distinguish this usage from the stricter one intended in this book, the adjective essential is occasionally added to the word nutrient to emphasise its specific meaning.

Strictly, nutrients are chemical components of food which are essential to life and health. These include the components which are used for the production of energy and the maintenance of metabolic function. Oxygen is not normally classed as a nutrient although it is absolutely essential for human life. Again, energy is not a nutrient in itself but is derived from a number of nutrients with the help of oxygen and is usefully considered as essential in its own right.

It is logical therefore to include bulk nutrients, organic nutrients, inorganic nutrients, water, oxygen and even energy itself under the banner of 'nutrients' in any discussion of human nutrition. In this book these will be considered in order of their gross daily requirements by the body.

Water is required in the greatest amount followed closely by oxygen. Among the nutrients, the amount of water actually in the body is also the greatest. On the other hand, the amount of free oxygen in the human body at any given time is relatively small. This is because oxygen is being continuously used up by the cells in metabolism. Both water and oxygen are the most urgently important substances for maintaining life.

All the remaining nutrients may be classified under two main headings namely energy providing nutrients and non-energy providing nutrients. Carbohydrates, lipids and proteins constitute the energy sources whereas the minerals and vitamins do not provide energy. The energy containing nutrients and the bulk minerals also give rise to the structural components in the body. The trace minerals and the vitamins are not normally considered as structural components although at the molecular level they are integral components of many systems such as enzymes.

Apart from water and oxygen all the remaining groups consist of a number of distinct nutrients and each of them is essential in its own right for maintaining human life. Throughout this book each nutrient will be considered in a separate chapter. Science has come a long way from the original Greek concept of four basic elements, namely water, air, fire and earth. From the nutritional point of view water is still water. Air contains oxygen which can be considered along with the other nutrients. Fire is not a nutrient as such but may be represented by the energy which food provides. And finally earth appropriately represents all the remaining nutrients required by the body.

There is considerable variation in nutrient intake from day to day. Table 2.1 gives examples of average daily nutrient intakes for several groups of people. The total intake may vary considerably but the overall distribution of different nutrients is less variable.

Table 2.1. Examples of daily nutrient intakes (all values in grams)

Nutrient group	Excessive intake	Typical man	Typical woman	Basic maintenance
Water	4,000	3,000	2,500	1,500
Oxygen	1,200	900	600	450
Carbohydrates	500	360	240	180
Lipids	200	120	80	60
Proteins	130	90	60	50
Minerals	50	35	25	15
Vitamins	trace	trace	trace	trace

The water values include the metabolic water of food but does not take account of sweating which can dramatically increase the requirement. The total carbohydrate should include around 20 to 30 grams of dietary fibre. The lipid should include around 15 grams of essential fatty acids and some authors claim that the protein should include around 1 gram of nucleic acids. The vitamin value would normally be less than one gram, probably in the range 100 to 300 milligrams, unless taking supplements.

3

Body Composition and Nutrients

The standard man weighs 70 kg (around 11 stone), has a height of 175 cm (5 foot 9 inches), uses up around 11,500 kJ (3,000 kcal) per day and is probably around 25 years of age. The standard woman weighs 58 kg (around 9 stone), has a height of 165 cm (5 foot 5 inches) uses up 9,500 kJ (2,300 kcal) and is also around 25 years old.

Such standards are arbitrary physiological references. Several sources use lighter adult standards of 65 kg for men and 55 kg for women, respectively. For example, one definition of a standard man is a man of 25 years, healthy, weight 65 kg, living in a temperate zone with a mean annual temperature of 10°C, and assumed to require an average daily intake of 13,500 kJ (or 3,200 kcal) of energy. The corresponding definition of a standard woman is a woman of 25 years, healthy, weight 55 kg, engaged in light industry or general household duties, living in a temperate zone with a mean annual temperature of 10°C, and assumed to require an average daily intake of 9,700 kJ (or 2,300 kcal) of energy.

Although each factor can vary independently, a clear relationship between weight and height is evident. Furthermore, tables of weights, which are widely used, are always related to heights. For both sexes, the weight and height should remain fairly constant throughout adult life. But, in reality, weight tends to increase with age up to about 50 years. Because of this fact, it is becoming more widespread to refer to actual median weights rather than standard weights for most nutritional purposes. Energy requirement however, decreases gradually with age. In many respects, a typical adult may be any age between about 24 and 50 years. Before 24 years of age an individual is still growing and after 50 (especially for women) further changes occur. Certainly, by the age of 75 the energy requirement has reduced significantly even in the healthiest of elderly persons. Table 3.1 summarises several characteristics so far discussed. The metabolic rate will be considered again in chapter 6.

Irrespective of weight, the human body is composed of a number of different organs and tissues. The most variable of these is the adipose or fat-containing tissue The 70 kg standard man contains muscle, fat bone, skin, blood, and so on as illustrated in Table 3.2. Apart from being generally smaller, women have a similar composition. However, when expressed as a percentage it can be seen that the typical woman has more lipid (or fat) and consequently less water than the typical man. Such composition expressed as a percentage of the principle nutrient groups is given in Table 3.3. This is often nutritionally more useful than purely anatomical details.

Table 3.1. Some factors of standard adults

Factor	Man	Woman
Weight	70 kg	58 kg
Height	175 cm	165 cm
Metabolic rate	12,500 kJ/day	9,500 kJ/day
	(3,000 cal/day)	(2,300 cal/day)
Surface area	1.85 sq.m	1.65 sq.m
Age	25 years	25 years

The average age of the US population is about 38 years. Adult men on average weigh about 79 kg and are 176 cm in height, whereas adult women on average weigh 63 kg and are 162 cm in height. Average weight and height varies from country to country.

Table 3.2. The standard male
(all values in kilograms)

Organ / Tissue	Weight
Muscle	27.0
Adipose tissue	12.0
Bone (total)	10.0
Skin (total)	6.5
Alimentary tract (total)	2.5
Liver	1.7
Brain	1.5
Lungs (both)	1.0
Lymphoid tissue	0.7
Heart	0.3
Kidneys (both)	0.3
Miscellaneous	1.0
Grand total	70.0

Table 3.3. Approximate composition of the standard human body

COMPONENT (nutrient group)	CONTENT (percent by weight)	
	Male	Female
Water	64	55
Oxygen	trace	trace
Carbohydrates	1	1
Lipids	14	25
Proteins	17	15
Minerals	4	4
Vitamins	trace	trace

4

Water

Common Name

Water.

Alternative Names

Liquids.
Fluids.
Drinks (somewhat incorrectly).

Nature

Water is a liquid with the formula H_2O. One litre of water weighs one kilogram approximately, in other words, every ml of water weighs almost exactly 1 g.

Requirement

The necessity of water has been known since the dawn of history. Water is one of the most important and least obvious of the nutrients. Anything from one-half to two-thirds of the total weight of the human body is water. People with large amounts of fat have a lower percentage of water than thin people. Women generally have a lower water content than men. The overall whole body composition was given in Table 3.3, in the previous chapter. Discounting the lipid, which is highly variable, both men and women have approximately the same water content in the remaining tissues, namely about 70 percent. The figures given in the table are for average men and women and should not imply that women are fatter than men. They do imply, however, that a woman naturally has a greater fat content than a man. This is a physiological fact of life. Consequently, women generally do have a lower water content than men. The daily requirement for water depends on a number of factors that influence the loss of water from the body. The most important of these are the temperature and humidity of the environment and the degree of physical activity, particularly if sweating occurs. Even in a cool environment without physical exertion a minimum amount of water is lost each day. The main losses occur in the urine, through the skin, in air exhaled from the lungs, and in the faeces. Sweating in particular can dramatically increase loss of water and salts. For example, a volume of fluid equal to the entire normal daily loss can occur in a single hour of profuse sweating. This sweating which occurs through the sweat glands can exceed 10 litres per day in certain circumstances. Water has a high heat capacity and latent heat of evaporation. For every gram (or ml) of water that is lost by evaporation the body loses 2.2 kilojoules (kJ) or about half of one kilocalorie (kcal). Thus the body loses at least one quarter of its total heat production in this way.

Even in the absence of sweating, traces of water slowly evaporate through the skin. This is called insensible perspiration because it is not normally noticed, yet it amounts to about 600 grams per day. By far the greatest loss occurs in the urine however, and only traces are lost in the faeces. These values are summarised in Table 4.1. The daily intake of water must balance the daily losses, and this balance is controlled exactly by thirst. Water is gained in three ways. It is usually taken in the largest quantity as fluid in drinks. It also occurs in wet food. And it occurs indirectly as the metabolic water of oxidised foods in the body during metabolism. Metabolic water will be further considered in the chapters on energy. Suffice it to say here that the metabolic water derived from food depends somewhat on its composition. For every 100 grams of pure substance the following water is produced: Carbohydrate gives rise to 56 g, lipid gives 107 g, protein gives 41 g and pure alcohol gives 117 g, respectively. The typical daily pattern of net gain and loss of water is summarised in Table 4.1.

There are several ways of estimating water requirement. One method allows a fixed quantity of water for each unit of energy used. In this way it can be shown that about 24 g water is required for every 100 kJ energy used in adults. In infants this allowance should be increased by fifty percent to 36 g per 100 kJ. Water is sometimes related to the total surface area of the body. Standard values of surface area were included in Table 3.2. The minimum requirement for adults is about 900 grams per square metre. The average is about 1,500 and the maximum tolerance is about 2,700 g per sq. m, respectively. These figures are only of academic interest, however. The overall obligatory (minimum) daily water requirement in adults is about 1,300 g and the optimum range is anywhere from about 2,000 to 4,000 g. The upper limit is around 5,000 g, not counting an allowance for sweating which can double or treble the daily requirement. Since most of the water in the diet comes directly from fluid drinks, and since the intake is controlled precisely by thirst, it is irrelevant here to include tables of the water content of various foodstuffs.

Toxicity

It is possible though extremely rare to drink enough water in a short time to cause death. About 8 to 10 litres in excess could cause death. Five litres (10 pints) of water would be quite nauseous whereas heavy drinkers can readily take ten pints of beer in the course of an evening. Part of the explanation is that the alcohol in the drink acts as a diuretic and speeds up the turnover. Water itself is non-toxic. However, in excess, its effect in the body is to cause water-logging (oedema), a dilution of the tissue salts such as sodium (hyponatremia) and possibly high blood pressure. A slowing of the heart rate may also occur. Serious effects include increased intracranial pressure, confusion, seizures, coma or even death.

Deficiency

Thirst is the first response to dehydration. There is a concentration of salts in the blood and tissues due to the loss of water. If sweating occurs at the same time, there is a loss of water and salts. A loss of only 2 percent body water results in thirst. Lack of water can result in renal failure. The blood becomes thicker and blood pressure increases. A buildup of toxins can occur accompanied by skin disorders. Cholesterol synthesis may increase. It has been argued that fat people can survive water depletion longer than thin people. This is because the metabolic water of fat is relatively high and they have more of it. A deficiency of water may also result in renal failure. If a person is deprived of water, severe dehydration occurs in a week or less depending on the temperature. When the total body water is reduced by 10 to 20 percent, or about 4 litres in all, death occurs.

Table 4.I. Water balance (all values in millilitres*)

DAILY GAIN OF WATER		DAILY LOSS OF WATER [a]	
Fluid drinks	1,400	Urine	1,500
Water in food	850	Evaporated from skin	550
Metabolic water	350	Expired from lungs	400
		Faeces	150
Net gain	2,600	Net loss	2,600

* One gram of water equals one millilitre, approximately.

a. Not counting sweating, if any.

5

Oxygen

Common Name

Oxygen.

Alternative Name

Air (incorrectly).

Nature

Oxygen is a gas with the formula O_2. It is found in air which consists of some 21 percent oxygen by volume. Every litre of air contains 210 ml oxygen which weighs 280 mg. Looking at this another way, one litre of pure oxygen weighs about 1.43 grams. Oxygen was discovered as a component of air by Lavoisier in 1774. Its importance to life was actually demonstrated one-hundred years earlier by Mayow who showed that a burning candle and a living mouse use up the same component of the air in a bell jar.

Requirement

Metabolism occurs in all cells in the body even when a person is asleep. The minimum obligatory metabolism is called basal metabolism and requires a certain minimum amount of oxygen. But a muscle can require up to fifty times more oxygen during vigorous activity. Table 5.1 shows how this may be achieved. During such periods of extra activity, the rate of respiration (breathing) is dramatically increased. This, together with the increased flow of blood to the limbs allows more oxygen to be extracted from the blood by the tissues.

The total amount of oxygen required is directly related to the overall energy expenditure of the individual. Energy is considered in more detail in the following three chapters. Although the element oxygen is widely distributed and occurs in the form of organic and inorganic components in food, the oxygen required by the body to produce energy, namely free oxygen, is absorbed from the air by the lungs. Oxygen is the only essential component required for life which is not obtained from food or drink. Each time we breath, about 400 ml of air is exchanged. About 250 ml of this reaches the alveoli deep in the lungs where the oxygen is absorbed and carbon dioxide is released. With extreme effort, it is possible to increase the volume of air exchanged in a single breath by a factor approaching 10. Although the alveoli are tiny, their great number means that the active surface area of the lungs is very large. The gas exchange area of the lungs has been estimated at 50 square metres and may be as great as 80 square meters in some individuals (the area of a circle approximately 60 feet in diameter).

In a typical 24-hour day, the total volume of air inhaled is around 20,000 litres. This contains 4,200 litres (or 6,000 grams) of pure oxygen, approximately, because air contains 21% pure oxygen. About 800 grams of this oxygen is actually absorbed by the lungs in a typical individual. The rate of breathing depends directly on the amount of oxygen required and is controlled by the brain.

At standard ambient temperature and pressure (25°C and one atmosphere pressure, 760 mmHg = 101.325 kPa), 1 mole of ideal gas has a volume of 24.466 litres. Therefore, oxygen (O_2), molar mass 32 g/mol, has a volume of 76.46 litres per 100 g. Typically, an adult requires around 400 to 500 grams (or 300 to 400 litres) of oxygen when using 6000 to 8000 kJ (or 1400 to 2000 kcal) energy per day.

For practical purposes, a general conversion factor may be used which relates 1 g oxygen used to every 14 kJ energy produced. In other words, every 20 kilojoules of bodily energy production requires one litre of oxygen intake, approximately.

Toxicity

Pure oxygen (which is five times more concentrated than the oxygen in the air) can be safely used for about 12 hours. After 24 hours, irritation of the lungs develops and there is a feeling of distress. The irritation of the lungs in this way can result in death. Excess oxygen in the tissues (hyperoxia) can cause cell damage including retinal damage. Oxygen under high pressure (as used by deep-sea divers) can only be used for short periods. At a pressure of several atmospheres convulsions may occur within a few hours. And after depressurisation there is another risk, namely the bends. The bends results from tiny bubbles of gas particularly nitrogen forming in the blood when the pressure is suddenly decreased after a long dive. To offset these effects divers sometimes substitute inert gasses such as helium, and keep the percentage of oxygen as low as possible. There are other risks with pressurised gas. At high pressure nitrogen acts as a narcotic, in other words it depresses the central nervous system.

Deficiency

All cells in the body require oxygen and the brain cannot survive for more than about four minutes at normal temperatures without it. Oxygen deficiency is termed anoxia. Irreversible damage may be caused even after a few minutes of deprivation. Deficiency of oxygen results in death.

Table 5.1. Supply of oxygen

SOURCE	MAXIMUM INCREASE (factor)
Blood flow rate	x 6
Redistribution of blood to muscles	x 3
Extraction from blood	x 3
Total increase	x 54

6

Energy Requirement

Common Names

Energy.
Activity.

Alternative Names

Metabolic energy.
Joules.
Work.
Heat.
Calories.

Nature

Energy is not a nutrient as such although it is essential for life. It is not a chemical either, although macronutrients in food contain chemical energy which is released when they are broken down in the body. Heat is a form of energy. In 1848, Joule was the first to establish that mechanical work (which is now measured in joules) and heat energy (which was previously measured in calories) are interchangeable. It is a matter of definition that 4.184 joules (J) equals 1 calorie (cal), exactly. This is the internationally accepted thermochemical conversion factor. For all practical purposes, however, 1 calorie is taken to equal 4.2 joules, approximately. Therefore 1,000 joules (or 1 kJ) equals 240 cal, approximately. In some books the large calorie (Cal) was used to represent a thousand small or ordinary calories (kcal). This usage is falling into decline. At present energy values are preferably quoted in joules. This unit was recommended for all forms of energy including food energy and metabolism, and it will eventually replace all the older calorie values. Commonly, energy values are now given in the new kJ units and equivalent values are quoted in calories for comparison.

Requirement

Our requirement for energy varies from hour to hour and from day to day. Each type of activity (or inactivity) requires a certain amount of metabolic energy. The overall expenditure of energy involves three components. In decreasing order of requirement, these are:

- Basal energy metabolism or resting energy expenditure (energy expended at rest)
- Physical activity (additional energy expended during physical activity)
- Thermogenesis (energy expended to produce heat in the body)

Table 6.1 lists ten high-energy activities and ten low-energy activities. Our typical daily routine probably contains a mixture of several of these activities. The typically daily energy expenditures for vigorously active lifestyles is around 17,000 kJ/d (~4,000 kcal/d), for moderately active lifestyles is around 12,500 kJ/d (~3,000 kcal/d) and for relatively inactive lifestyles is around 8,000 kJ/d (~2,000 kcal/d), respectively.

Excess

Energy is contained in several nutrients but is not itself a nutrient. Energy, in various forms, is all around us but is not available as metabolic energy other than through eating food. Within limits, most forms of energy do us no harm. An excessive intake of food energy results in a gain of weight. This will be considered again in the chapter on lipids. There is a disease of the thyroid gland called hypothyroidism, a deficiency of thyroid hormones, which results in the depression of energy utilisation. In these cases, there is a general lowering of the basal metabolic rate and an overall gain in weight. In many respects this is analogous to an excessive intake of energy.

Deficiency

A deficiency of energy intake relative to bodily expenditure over a long period of time will result in a loss of weight. This is a result of the body having to use up its own stores (principally of fat but eventually of protein as well) to provide the required energy. Many factors influence basal metabolism and this varies from individual to individual. As a first approximation, the following values based on overall surface area (of the skin) are sometimes used: 170 kJ (40 kcal) per square meter per hour for men and 155 (37 kcal) per square meter per hour for women, respectively. These do not take additional activities into account after reaching full maturity. There is a gradual decrease in overall energy requirement as we grow older. Injury and stress may increase the requirement for energy. An excessively high rate of utilisation of energy can also occur in another disease of the thyroid gland called thyrotoxicosis. Here the body energy stores are broken down at a faster rate than they are required. This results in a loss of weight. The disease is accompanied by numerous unpleasant sensations resulting in a general nervousness. The excessive breakdown of body energy is in many ways analogous to an overall deficiency of energy. Continued starvation results in death usually after about six to ten weeks, provided only water is taken.

Table 6.1. The energy cost of various activities
(all values in joules per hour)

HIGH ENERGY ACTIVITIES		LOW ENERGY ACTIVITIES	
Handball	2,560	Bowling; Bed-making;	1,000
Skiing	2,480	Walking; Scrubbing floors	900
Riding horseback	2,000	Preparing a meal	830
Lawn mowing by hand	1,930	Driving a car	700
Farm field work	1,850	Standing up	570
Sawing; Carpentry	1,750	Sweeping; Cleaning	530
Ballroom dancing	1,380	Deskwork; Painting at easel	500
Walking down Stairs	1,300	Sitting knitting; Eating	370
Swimming; Golf	1,250	Sitting; Reading	300
Ironing, standing up	1,100	Sleeping (basal)	250

It may help to compare the new energy units with the old by giving a practical example. An ordinary 100-watt light bulb radiates 360 kJ energy in the form of light and heat per hour. Over a period of one day, if the bulb is left on, it radiates the equivalent of about 2,000 kcal, which is the typical daily energy output of an individual. Put another way, the metabolic energy produced by a typical adult could keep a 100-watt bulb lighting indefinitely.

7

Energy Metabolism

Every mouthful of food contains energy (calories). Energy metabolism is the study of the conversion of food into energy in the body. Just as when organic matter, in the form of coal, wood, turf or oil is burnt in air to produce heat; food in the form of carbohydrates, lipids or proteins is similarly used up in the body. This latter activity occurs much more slowly to provide heat and energy for the body. In both cases however, the basic elements of carbon, hydrogen and oxygen in the material are converted in the presence of additional oxygen into carbon dioxide and water.

For example, consider the complete combustion or metabolism of the carbohydrate glucose which has the chemical formula $C_6H_{12}O_6$. The reaction may be written as follows:

$$C_6H_{12}O_6 \ + \ 6\,O_2 \ = \ 6\,CO_2 \ + \ 6\,H_2O \ + \ kJ$$

Glucose   Oxygen   Carbon Dioxide   Water   Energy

In this equation, $C_6H_{12}O_6$ represents one molecule (or molar mass) of pure glucose (which is a solid). The O_2 and CO_2 are the gases, oxygen and carbon dioxide, which are exchanged in the lungs. For each molecule of glucose used up in the reaction, six molecules of oxygen are required and five molecules of carbon dioxide are produced. The five molecules of water also produced in this reaction represent the metabolic water of glucose. The metabolism of all foodstuffs results in the production of some water in this way. In Table 4.1 it was indicated that on average about 350 ml (or g) of water per day comes from food in this way. And, last but not least, the metabolism of foodstuffs releases chemical energy.

Typical chemical reactions for the other types of food molecules are as follows.

Mixture of lipids (oleic, palmitate and stearic acids):

$$C_{52}H_{104}O_6 + 75O_2 = 52CO_2 + 52H_2O + kJ$$

Typical protein:

$$C_{362}H_{586}N_{104}O_{104}S + 3800O_2 = 52H_2NCONH_2 + 310CO_2$$
$$+ 188H_2O + H_2SO_4 + kJ$$

Alcohol (ethanol):

$$C_2H_5OH + 3O_2 = 2CO_2 + 3H_2O + kJ$$

Suffice it to say that the amount of energy varies somewhat for different types of food and may be represented in a number of alternative ways as summarised in Table 7.1. These values vary from source to source because they depend also on the chemical nature of the test substrate used. For example, fatty acids of different composition (number of carbons) will have slightly different values, and so on. However, these differences are less important nutritionally than the digestibility factor.

Almost everyone interested in dieting knows that one gram of carbohydrate or protein yields 4 calories, whereas one gram of fat yields 9 calories. These are the traditionally used rounded average factors first used by Atwater at the turn of the last century, and are still regarded as accurate enough for most diets. In fact, different sources of carbohydrate, lipid and protein have slightly different values. These detailed values are more nutritionally relevant because they also take into account the degree of digestibility of a given source. To make this distinction clear, consider 100 g of carbohydrate from two different sources, A and B, respectively. Source A is easy to digest and gives virtually 100 percent energy value. Source B, on the other hand, is not so easily digested and therefore only a fraction of its total energy (say 75 percent) is available for utilisation. It can be concluded that 75 g of carbohydrate from source A gives the same amount of metabolisable energy as the full 100 g from source B. In other words, the energy yield from source A is higher than that from source B. In reality, the differences found are slight and are mainly of academic rather than of practical interest.

To make calculating easier for the energy (or calorie) conscious individual, values are not normally quoted per gram of each food component but per amount of the total food itself. Usually, the value of some convenient amount, representing a portion, is used. This leads to some confusion when comparing potions of different weight. Appendix A1 lists the gram and millilitre equivalents of a number of commonly used portions. The most useful portions however are 100 g for solid food and 100 ml for liquids. The density of liquids varies quite a lot, so it is not possible to assume that 100 ml equals 100 g except in a few cases.

Throughout this series, each nutrient will be listed in a compendium indicating its relative level in ten different food groups. The overall metabolisable energy values of the food groups is given in the first compendium of this type in Table 7.2. Further details on the food groups are given in Chapter 10.

Table 7.1. Energy values of food components

SUBSTANCE	ENERGY			
	Per gram of food metabolised kJ (kcal)		Per litre of oxygen consumed kJ (kcal)	
Carbohydrates	17.5	(4.2)	21.0	(5.0)
Lipids	39.0	(9.3)	19.5	(4.7)
Proteins	18.5	(4.4)	20.0	(4.8)
Alcohol	29.5	(7.1)	20.5	(4.9)
Organic Acids	10.5	(2.5)	19.0	(4.5)

It can be seen that the values expressed per gram vary markedly, whereas the values expressed per litre of oxygen consumed are very similar. A working average of 20 kJ (or 4.8 kcal) per litre of oxygen is often used in nutrition studies. The values for each gram of food are considered in more detail in the text.

General conversion factors, representing average values, may be used in most nutritional estimates. These are given as follows: lipids 38 kJ (9 kcal); alcohol 29 kJ (7 kcal); carbohydrates and proteins 17 kJ (4 kcal); organic acids 10 kJ (2.5 kcal) and dietary fibre and water nil.

Table 7.2. Energy Compendium

FOOD GROUP	ENERGY
Milk and products	Medium, variable
Eggs	Low
Meat / Fish	Medium / Low, variable
Fats and Oils	Very high
Grain and products	Medium, variable
Nuts / Pulses	Very high / Very low, variable
Root vegetables	Very low
Leaf vegetables	Very low
Fruit	Very low
Sweets	High

8

Energy and a Balanced Diet

Having considered typical daily requirement of energy and energy metabolism, it remains to describe how best to manage overall energy intake. As a general guide, one should maintain the same weight throughout adult life. There are risks to health of being too overweight or underweight. For example, if a person is considerably overweight it may be advisable to reduce the food intake per day and thus reduce weight. But rapid weight losses are not recommended. Consider the following calculation. One kilogram of adipose fat contains approximately 32,000 (or about 7,500 kcal) of metabolisable energy. The difference between this value and that given for pure fat is due to traces of other substances (notably about 10 % water) which are present in the adipose tissue. So by reducing the average weekly intake by this amount one should expect to lose about 1 kg per week. A steady weight loss of about 1 kg (or 2 pounds) per week is the safest way to go about dieting. This rate of progress should be achievable for most by reducing the daily energy intake by about 6,000 to 4,000 kJ depending on a number of factors. Generally, men can reduce their intake by up to 1,500 kcal (in old units) and women can reduce their intake by up to 1,000 kcal, for limited periods of time without serious risk. There are many foolish, if not downright dangerous, theories about dieting. Any diet that does not recommend a balanced intake of energy-providing nutrients is in error! But, simply from the point of view of providing useful energy, it makes little difference whether the bulk of our food intake is in the form of carbohydrate, lipid or protein (or indeed even alcohol). However, when other nutritional considerations are taken into account, it is important to have a proper balance between the main components.

Some well-known recommendations on human nutrition are summarised in Table 8.1. More details on various carbohydrates, lipids and proteins are given in the following chapters. Here, it is sufficient to note the overall balance. For every 100 kJ (or in this case, 100 kcal also), it is recommended that over one half (58 percent) should come from carbohydrate sources. The carbohydrates should furthermore, be of two types. Most of it should be of the rough or complex type and only a small portion should be of the simpler or refined type. Less than one third (30 percent) of our food should be in the form of lipid. Of this, one third should be of the saturated type, one third monounsaturated and one third polyunsaturated. These terms will be explained in the chapters on lipids. Regarding proteins, only about one-eight (12 percent) of our energy should come in this form. Again, proteins should be from mixed sources, generally about two-thirds should come from animal sources and one third from plant sources. Most Western diets contain about the right amount of protein, but perhaps less animal protein and more plant protein should be used. Regarding carbohydrates there is a widespread overuse of refined forms and not enough use of complex forms which include roughage (fibre). On the whole, if the complex form was increased and the refined form reduced, the balance would again be more appropriate. Finally, regarding the lipids, there is probably too little of the unsaturated form relative to the saturated form. Again, a slight overall decrease in fat intake would be beneficial in most cases.

The average percentage energy values contributed by carbohydrates, lipids and proteins in various food groups is given for comparison in Table 8.2. An ideal balance may best be achieved by suitable mixtures of different groups. There are many common sense rules of thumb which, if followed, provide perfectly adequate diets. Menu books are also a great help in planning sensible meals with balance and variety. Giving such advice, however, is an applied branch of nutrition and is outside the scope of this introductory book on the nutrients. Irrespective of the type of food, when there is continuous overeating, even of only a few grams per day, there will also be a continuous increase in weight. It can be estimated that an excess of only 500 kJ (about 120 kcal, or approximately 20 g of mixed food) per week will result in an increase of two and a half stone (about 16 kg) over a 20-year period. In most cases this is the explanation of so-called middle-aged spread. Fortunately, with determination, one can lose this extra weight over a much shorter period but preferably not shorter the three months. After the next chapters which deal with digestion and food (again), we will consider the three main groups of energy providing nutrients namely the carbohydrates, lipids and proteins, in more detail.

Table 8.1. A balanced intake of energy yielding foods
(as a percentage of total energy intake)

FOOD				TYPE
Carbohydrates	58	{	48	Complex
			10	Refined
Lipids	30	{	10	Fully saturated
			10	Monounsaturated
			10	Polyunsaturated
Proteins	12	{	8	Animal origin
			4	Plant origin

The above recommendation is based on "Dietary Goals for the United States", as suggested by the US Senate Select Committee on Nutrition and Human Needs, 2nd ed. US Government Printing Office (1977).

The Acceptable Macronutrient Distribution Ranges (AMDR)[1] may be summarised as follows. Around 45 to 65 percent of adult daily calories should come from carbohydrates, 10 to 35 percent from proteins, and 20 to 35 percent from total lipids, of which 5 to 10 percent should come from linoleic acid and 0.6 to 1.2 percent from α-linolenic acid. The guidelines also recommend that refined sugars should be limited to a maximum of 25 percent of total energy and that cholesterol, saturated fatty acids and trans fatty acids should be kept as low as possible in an adequate diet.

1. Dietary Reference Intakes for Energy, Carbohydrate, Fiber, Fat, Fatty Acids, Cholesterol, Protein, and Amino Acids (Macronutrients) (2005). Food and Nutrition Board of the Institute of Medicine in cooperation with Canadian scientists. The National Academies Press.

Table 8.2. Energy distribution pattern in various foods
(as percentages of total energy)

FOOD GROUP	ENERGY DISTRIBUTION		
	CARBOHYDRATES	LIPIDS	PROTEINS
Milk and products	29	48	23
Eggs	2	65	33
Meat and fish	0	68	32
Fats and oils	0	100	0
Grain and products	80	8	12
Nuts and pulses	33	48	20
Root vegetables	88	1	10
Leaf vegetables	78	7	15
Fruit	93	3	4
Sweets	100	0	0

Some food groups have considerable variation. For example, cheeses vary considerable and, in general, have higher protein and lipid and lower carbohydrate than milk. Certain meats and oily fish have higher lipid content. Nuts in general also have a higher lipid content than pulses.
The zero in some columns may imply trace values.

9

Digestion

All the nutrients described in this book (except the essential substance, oxygen) enter the body through the alimentary tract. Before considering individual nutrients in detail it may be helpful to briefly consider digestion in general.

The process of digestion starts in the mouth, where food is mixed with a neutral secretion called saliva before being swallowed. Over one litre of saliva is produced per day. Apart from providing lubrication saliva also contains an enzyme called amylase which helps to break down complex carbohydrates called starches and glycogens. The action of amylase does not last long. In less than a minute, as a rule, food is swallowed and enters the most acidic fluid in the body namely gastric juice, in the stomach.

The acid conditions in the stomach continue the processes of digestion of many complex components in food. Foods with a high fat content remain longest in the stomach. And food in general may remain in the stomach for several hours whereas liquids tend to pass through rapidly. The average delay in the stomach is about hour. Apart from the acid known as hydrochloric acid, gastric juice also contains enzymes. One of these enzymes called pepsin helps to break down some proteins. In infants an additional enzyme called rennin helps to curdle milk.

On leaving the stomach the food enters the upper small intestine or duodenum where it is mixed with an alkaline secretion called pancreatic juice. Approximately 1.3 litres of pancreatic juice is produced per day. This juice neutralises the stomach acid and contains a variety of enzymes which continue to act on various food components. An enzyme called pancreatic amylase continues breaking down the remaining starches. Trypsin, chymotrypsin and carboxypeptidase continue to break down the remaining protein fragments. An enzyme called lipase breaks down lipids. There are several enzymes that act on other components for example the cholesterol related lipids and the nucleic acids. All the above mentioned enzymatic processes continue throughout the small intestine. While in the small intestine food is also mixed with the digestive juice called bile which is formed in the liver and stored in the gall bladder. Bile contains emulsifying agents which break up various fat globules into smaller fragments. About 0.7 litres (700 ml) of bile is produced per day. Also the small intestine itself contributes a copious secretion containing many additional enzymes which supplement the work of digestion already begun. About 3 litres of intestinal juice is produced per day. Its enzymes include sucrase which breaks down table sugar, lactase which breaks down milk sugar, phosphatase which frees phosphates, and many others. Food remains in the small intestine for about 4 hours altogether.

The final stages of digestion occur in the large intestine or colon. Here a large number of different bacteria assist in breaking down most of the remaining material. The last of the food components are absorbed there including most of the remaining water and salts. The residue thus formed is expelled approximately once a day in the faeces. These consist of indigestible fibre, dead cells and bacteria, and all of the unabsorbed components of food breakdown. The daily faecal mass is about 100 to 250 grams per day. In general, the greater the dietary fibre intake the greater the faecal output. Table 9.1 summarises some data on the gastro-intestinal tract.

Various nutrients may either be absorbed by simple passive processes or by active mechanisms which involve transport carriers to ferry the nutrients into the cell. Such considerations need not concern us here. Carbohydrates, free amino acids and some lipid components are absorbed directly into the blood stream whereas other components such as the lipids in general are first taken up in the lymph and only thereafter enter the blood. Vitamins are absorbed in two different ways. The water soluble vitamins are absorbed directly into the blood whereas the fat soluble vitamins tend to accompany the other lipids into the lymph. The minerals in general tend to be absorbed directly into the blood, also. There is very little absorption from the mouth or from the stomach with the notable exception of alcohol itself. The small intestine is without a doubt the main organ of digestion and absorption. Up to 90 percent of the total nutrient intake is absorbed there. Finally, most of the water (including the water contributed by the digestive secretions, and their salts) is absorbed in the large intestine.

Table 9.1. Some data on the gastro-intestinal tract

ORGAN	Approximate volume of digestive secretions (litres per day)	Mass of local contents (grams)	Average time food remains therein (hours)
Mouth	1.2	negligible	negligible
Stomach	2.5	250	1
Small intestine *	5.0	1,200	4
Large intestine	trace	300	18

* Total including bile, pancreatic juice and intestinal juice.

10

Food

There are many ways of classifying food. For this purposes of this book it will be convenient to use ten major groups. In various chapters a compendium table summarises the relative abundance of each nutrient in these ten categories. For each class of food, the overall (average) nutrient level is indicated on a simple score as follows: very high, high, medium, low, very low or nil (negligible). These are intended to be broad classifications and in all but a few cases do not include exceptions. More detailed figures are however included in the high- and low- tables. In these tables ten very high or high and ten very low or nil foods are listed together with estimates of their content. Again, the information is not exhaustive or absolute, and the examples given are selected from a wide variety of sources. Only common foods or food products are included. Special supplements or very rare and exotic foods are excluded. Brand products are also omitted. It should be pointed out, however, that the actual value of the food that arrives on our plate is dependent on its full history up to that point. Cooking for example destroys varying amounts of vitamin activity while making other components more digestible. The values given are therefore for food as usually eaten and include a correction for cooking (average time) where such losses occur.

The ten major food groups are as follows:

- Milk and its products
- Eggs
- All meat including poultry,
- and fish including shellfish
- Fats and oils

- Grain (cereals) and its products

- Nuts and pulses (legumes)

- Root vegetables

- Leaf vegetables

- Fruit

- Sweets

Each group will now be briefly considered.

Milk and its Products

Milk is obtained from several sources but particularly the cow. Milk is a moderate source of energy and contains all the major nutrients required for growth and maintenance except perhaps iron, copper and vitamin C. Products such as cream and cheese are fractions rich in lipid or protein respectively, although cheeses vary considerably in composition. Milk is rich in carbohydrate, lipid and protein. Milk sugar is called lactose and the principle milk protein is casein which is a complete protein containing all the essential amino acids. Milk is a major source of the minerals calcium and phosphorous and contains traces of other minerals such as potassium. Milk also contains vitamins particularly the B complex vitamins and vitamin D. Cheeses are generally richer in protein and possibly lipid than milk itself. Yoghurts are generally higher in Vitamins and lower in lipid than milk but brands vary considerably. Butter is a product of milk, but is classified in a separate group being virtually 100 percent lipid. On the other hand, dried skimmed milk is generally low in lipid.

Eggs

Eggs are low in energy. They contain little carbohydrate but are a rich source of lipid (including cholesterol) and complete protein. The principle vitamins include several of the B complex and the fat soluble vitamins A, D and E. Eggs may be separated into the white and the yolk. The white is virtually pure protein called albumen with traces of minerals and vitamins. The yolk is a rich source of lipids including the phospholipids making them the richest known source of choline. The lipids contain a high percentage of unsaturated fatty acids and also include a very high content of cholesterol. The yolk also contains a rich source of protein (including nucleic acids).

Meat and Fish

Meat and fish are moderate sources of energy. They contain virtually no carbohydrate but are excellent sources of lipid and protein. The amount of fat varies considerably. Pork is the highest in lipid and contains three times more energy than most other cuts of meat. All visible fat is likewise almost pure lipid. On the other hand, even the leanest cut of meat contains some lipid. In general poultry and fish are markedly low in energy. Fish itself varies, for example, oily fish such as salmon are higher in lipid than white fish. Fish in general are good sources of polyunsaturated fatty acids. Shellfish also contain moderate amounts of cholesterol but are low in other lipids. Meat and fish are excellent sources of complete protein and also contain a variety of important minerals and vitamins. The fat soluble vitamins are associated with the fatty types of meat and fish. Organ meats such as liver and kidney are excellent sources of many elements and vitamins, including iron and phosphorous, the B vitamin complex and vitamins C, and the fat soluble vitamins A and D. Processed meat such as pies and sausages have less protein and considerable quantities of fat. Fish is an important source of the trace elements iodine and vanadium. Freshwater fish contain traces of magnesium, iron and copper. Salt-water fish contain traces of fluorine and cobalt in addition to iodine and shellfish contain zinc.

Fats and Oils

Fats and oils are the richest source of lipid (and consequently energy) and associated nutrients such as the fat-soluble vitamins. Animal fats contain mainly saturated lipid whereas plant oils are a valuable source of unsaturated lipids. Pure fats and oils are devoid of carbohydrate and protein. They do however contain a number of minerals in trace amounts.

Grain and its Products

Grain is a moderate source of energy. Grain contains complex carbohydrates is a major component. Whole grains are an important source of dietary fibre which although indigestible nevertheless aids the function of the alimentary tract. Grain is low in lipid and protein, which is incomplete. Whole grains are a good source of the B complex vitamins and contain a range of minerals and trace elements. A typical wheat grain is made up of a covering called bran (about 14 percent), a germ or growing part (about 3 percent) and the main (flour) part called the endosperm (about 83 percent). The bran containing dietary fibre and much of the vitamins is usually discarded. The germ containing much of the remaining vitamins is also removed before making flour for white bread. The remaining endosperm consists of starch and protein and contains only a fraction of the total vitamin value. Grain products include a wide variety of food such as breakfast cereals, bread of various types and rice. In general grain products are deficient in the fat-soluble vitamins although traces of vitamin A and are present in the germ. Vitamin C is also absent from grain. Grain is deficient in the essential amino acid lysine. In addition, maize (corn) is also deficient in tryptophan, another essential amino acid.

Nuts and Pulses

Nuts are an excellent source of energy. They are generally rich in carbohydrate, lipid and protein. Seeds such as sunflower seeds are included in this group and are very rich in lipid (oil) of the unsaturated type. Nuts contain a number of minerals such as calcium and phosphorous, potassium and iron. Nuts are a good source of several vitamins such as the B complex and Vitamin E. An interesting feature of nuts and pulses is their high quality protein which includes lysine (the amino acid deficient in grain). The protein is not quite complete and is low in the essential amino acid methionine. Pulses are a moderate source of energy. Pulses are leguminous seeds and include various peas, beans and lentils. They also include peanuts (ground nuts). Like nuts they are an excellent source of carbohydrates and proteins, though in general have less lipid. They are similar in overall nutritive value to nuts. Sprouted pulses are richer in certain vitamins, including vitamin C, than unsprouted seeds. In general nuts and pulses have a good balance of minerals and trace elements.

Root Vegetables

Roots are a poor source of energy. The edible roots include potatoes, sweat potatoes, carrots, turnips and parsnips. They are an excellent source of complex carbohydrate, have some protein but little lipid. Generally, they are low in minerals and vitamins but there are some exceptions. For example, carrots are an excellent source of β-carotene (a vitamin A precursor). However, when taken in quantity they are a valuable source of minerals in the diet.

Leaf Vegetables

Leaf vegetables are a very poor source of energy. They are an excellent source of complex carbohydrate relative to their lipid and protein content. The quality of the protein in most plant foods is poorer than that from animal sources. However, when eaten in bulk they contribute to the protein to the diet. Green and yellow vegetables contain β-carotene, Vitamin C and several of the B complex vitamins. They also contain a range of mineral including calcium, iron and potassium. Tomatoes and cucumbers may be included in this category.

Fruit

Fruit is a poor source of energy with a few exceptions such as the banana and all dried fruit. Fruit is the richest source of carbohydrates (if sweets are excluded) on a percentage basis. Fruit also contains a variety of minerals and vitamins. Apples and bananas for example contain dietary fibre. Fruit, particularly the citrus varieties such as oranges, lemons, grapefruit and tangerines, are rich sources of vitamin C. Yellow fruits also contain β-carotene. Bananas are a good source of magnesium. Many fruits also contain simple sugars, for example bananas and pears. Fruit juices may be included in this group.

Sweets

Sweets include sugars, soft drinks, candies and sweet desserts. Sweets are a high source of energy because they contain concentrated simple sugars, such as sucrose and very little else. They are practically devoid of all other nutrients. Even natural sweeteners such as honey only contain traces of minerals and vitamins (which are nutritionally insignificant!) Table sugar is essentially pure crystalline sucrose. Chocolate and cocoa contain large counts of carbohydrates. Honey, treacle, syrup and molasses are all forms of sugar which contain traces of minerals and vitamins and water. Saccharine is a sugar substitute that does not contribute to the energy intake in the diet.

11

Carbohydrates (and Organic Acids)

Common Name

Carbohydrates.

Alternative Names

Carbs.
Sugars and Starches.
Mono-, di- and poly- saccharides.
Hexoses and Pentoses.

The following are specific compounds:

Glucose, Fructose, Galactose, Ribose,
Sucrose, Maltose and Lactose.
Glycogen.

Nature

Carbohydrate is a conditionally essential nutrient. All carbohydrates are made up of basic units called monosaccharides. The most representative carbohydrate unit is called glucose. Glucose contains six carbon atoms, six oxygen atoms and twelve hydrogen atoms. Hence the formula $C_6H_{12}O_6$, which is commonly used to represent the carbohydrates. Carbohydrates may be defined chemically as polyhydroxy aldehydes or ketones. Starch is made up of straight chains and glycogen is made up of branched chains of glucose molecules joined together. Starches are the main plant polysaccharide whereas glycogen is the main animal form. The body is able to synthesise glucose and convert carbohydrates into other materials notably lipids. Carbohydrates may be divided into four main groups as follows:

- monosaccharides (single sugars) such as glucose, fructose and ribose,

- disaccharides (double sugars) such as sucrose, lactose and maltose,

- polysaccharides (multiple or complex carbohydrates) such as starch, glycogen, dextrin and dietary fibre.

The first three groups represent the available carbohydrate. The first two groups are simple sugars and usually taste sweet. The third group includes the complex carbohydrates which are available for absorption after being broken down to free glucose during digestion. The last represents the unavailable or indigestible carbohydrate, and includes various pectins, gums, celluloses and lignin. Very high-fibre foods are therefore somewhat lower in energy than non-fibrous foods of otherwise similar composition. However, dietary fibre is absent from many foods. A separate chapter on dietary fibre follows this chapter.

Biological Functions

- Although the dietary intake of carbohydrate is generally the greatest of all the food nutrients, only traces are found stored in the body. This is because the major role of the carbohydrates is to provide energy for day-to-day activities. The total carbohydrate in the body is equivalent to only 10,000 to 12,000 kJ (about one day's supply of energy).

- Carbohydrate helps regulate the metabolism of protein and lipids, and may be stored in the form of glycogen in liver and muscle.

- Many amino acids can give rise to glucose. These are called glucogenic amino acids, and represent an important alternative source of energy. Up to 60 percent of dietary protein may lend itself to conversion in this way under certain circumstances.

- A small amount of carbohydrate is necessary to spare wasteful protein metabolism in the body.

- Nonessential amino acids may be interconverted with the aid of carbohydrate derivatives in the body.

- Glycerol, a lipid component, may give rise to small amounts of glucose when necessary (for example during periods of fasting).

- An excess of carbohydrate is converted to fat in the body.

- Small amounts of carbohydrate limit the breakdown of lipid and prevent ketosis (which is an excessive production of ketones due to rapid fat breakdown).

Requirement

In the body, carbohydrates may be derived from either the glucogenic amino acids or the glycerol component of certain lipids. Therefore, there is strictly no absolute minimum requirement for carbohydrate intake provided that adequate amounts of protein and fat are consumed. Otherwise, it is found that a complete absence of dietary carbohydrate results in excessive breakdown of fats and causes ketosis.

The recommended daily intake is around 130 g for adults. Average intakes greatly exceed these values in some cases, though the excesses are generally not as great as with lipid intake. A carbohydrate compendium lists the relative abundance of total carbohydrate in various food groups (Table 11.1). The best sources of carbohydrates include sugar itself, honey, jams, biscuits bread, chocolate, cakes and doughnuts.

Toxicity

Excessive carbohydrate intake may overload the insulin control system and potentiate diabetes. Continued excessive intake results in an increase in weight, but in general carbohydrates are non-toxic. An excess of carbohydrate, particularly glucose (hyperglycemia), can result in coma.

Deficiency

Prolonged deficiency of carbohydrate results in a loss of weight. A specific deficiency of carbohydrate (hypoglycemia) will result in ketosis. The glucose level in the blood must be kept within certain levels. Very high or very low levels can result in coma, and risk of death if not corrected quickly.

Organic Acids

In addition to the carbohydrates, the organic acids may also be mentioned in this chapter. Organic acids are not essential nutrients and are negligible in most foods. They do however occur in small quantities in certain fruit and vegetables where they can contribute up to 6 and 12 percent, respectively, of the total metabolisable energy value.

The two most important organic acids are citric acid and malic acid. These are not essential because they can be produced during the breakdown of carbohydrates in the body. The best sources of organic acids include lemon juice, grapefruit, cranberries, oranges, plumbs and squash. The organic acid content of most other foods is negligible. Lemon juice is an interesting exception. Over 60 percent of its energy derives from organic acids. Nevertheless, its overall contribution to dietary energy, even when taken in large quantities is small. This is because the total energy value of lemon juice is so small.

Table 11.1. Carbohydrate Compendium

FOOD GROUP	CARBOHYDRATE LEVEL
Milk and products	Low, variable
Eggs	Low
Meat and fish	Nil
Fats and oils	Nil
Grain and products	Very high
Nuts and pulses	High
Roof vegetables	Medium
Leaf vegetables	Medium
Fruit	Medium
Sweets	Very high

Table 11.2. Contribution of organic acids to total energy value of selected foods.

FOOD	CONTRIBUTION (percent of total energy)
FRUIT	
Lemon Juice	62.5
Grapefruit	11.3
Cranberries	9.6
Oranges	6.5
Plums	6.0
Prunes	5.9
Pineapple	4.2
VEGETABLES	
Squash	12.3
Cauliflower	6.5
Tomatoes	6.2
Kale	3.6
Lettuce	3.5
Brussels sprouts	3.2
Carrots	2.8
Cabbage	2.3

The total energy value of lemon juice is only about 100 kJ per 100 ml, so, even in this unusual case, the organic acid contribution to the dietary energy intake is negligible.

12

Dietary Fibre

Common Name

Dietary Fibre.

Alternative Names

Crude Fibre (incorrectly).
Roughage.
Indigestible Fibre, or simply fibre.
Unavailable carbohydrate. Non-starch polysaccharide.
Bran.

Nature

For years dietary fibre was completely ignored. Now the tables have turned, and it is the subject of intensive study which is pointing to some unusual and exciting results. The prime movers in this new phase were Burkitt, Cleave and Trowell who began to look at the subject in the sixties. The term dietary fibre was first used specifically in 1972 by Trowell.

The complex carbohydrates include glycogen (animal polysaccharide) and starch and dietary fibre (plant polysaccharides). In contrast to the simple sugars they do not taste sweet, and they take longer to digest. Dietary fibre itself is indigestible but has an important function in regulating the movement of the bowel. As a general rule, dietary fibre is found in association with other complex carbohydrates of plant origin. Dietary fibre consists of cellulose, hemicellulose, pectins, gums, alginates (all of which are carbohydrates) and lignins and cutins (which are non-carbohydrate).

Crude fibre, which is the residue left after chemical hydrolysis consists mainly of cellulose, hemicellulose and some lignin. Dietary fibre, therefore, contains a number of additional components. It is theoretically possible for some bacteria in the large intestine to break down fibre slightly, but this is of limited nutritional significance. Older food tables gave values for crude fibre. Newer tables, give the more relevant dietary fibre values which are somewhat larger than the older crude fibre values.

Biological Functions

- Dietary fibre regulates the movement of the bowel. It influences all parts of the digestive system but particularly the small and large intestine. Dietary fibre is hygroscopic, that is it absorbs water, and hence it helps to soften and assist the normal elimination of the faeces.

- A diet rich in fibre is correspondingly lower in energy (particularly sugar and lipid) and satisfies hunger at lower energy intakes. This results in a tendency to eat less and is one way to prevent obesity.

- Dietary fibre may absorb dietary cholesterol and thereby help to reduce its level in the circulation.

- Dietary fibre may protect the large intestine from certain toxins by absorbing and eliminating them. Also, because of the increased bulk of the faeces, dietary fibre may dilute potential carcinogens especially in the large intestine and colon.

- Dietary fibre may protect against a number of apparently diverse diseases. These are considered in the final section of this chapter.

Requirement

The normal adult should consume at least 25 grams of fibre per day. The average intake in the Western diet is about half this level. Desirable levels have been estimated at between 30 and 40 grams per day for adult males and between 20 and 25 grams per day for adult females. Probably, 75 grams per day is an upper limit. Infants apparently do not need fibre. A dietary fibre compendium is included for information (Table 12.1). As a general rule, only plant foods contain dietary fibre. The best sources of dietary fibre include bran, whole grain products, nuts, peas, lentils, dried dates and raisins. It is recommended to increase dietary fibre by eating more whole grain products, pulses, vegetables and fruit for example, rather than by simply increasing the intake of fibre supplements. It is also recommended to leave the skin on fruits and vegetables, as it is high in fiber.

Toxicity

Fibre is essentially non-toxic. Excessive intake dramatically increases faecal output. It may cause distension of the gut with discomfort due to excessive gas production (flatulence). Excessive intakes may also deplete certain nutrients by adsorption, particularly the minerals calcium, magnesium, iron and zinc. There may be a feeling of nausea which may prompt vomiting in some cases. Fibre tends to reduce low-density lipoprotein (LDL) cholesterol. Excessive fibre may also cause dehydration.

Deficiency

In the West, ten times more refined carbohydrates and three times more lipid (mainly of animal origin) is consumed than in the Third World. On the other hand, three times less dietary fibre is consumed. This results in a number of adverse effects. Dietary fibre is not strictly a nutrient in the traditional sense of the word. But the term nutrient should ideally include all beneficial substances, even those that are not digested or absorbed. Oxygen has already been included as a nutrient on the grounds that it is essential for life, although it is not obtained free as such in food. A case can also be made for sunlight (in connection with the vitamin D story). Dietary fibre is a component of some foods and although it may not be absolutely essential for life, its absence results in various bowel disturbances and may, it seems, lead to several debilitating diseases.

People in the Third World consume 40 – 60 grams of dietary fibre per day whereas, in the West, the normal intake is only 15 – 25 grams per day and a number of diseases rarely found elsewhere are commonplace.

Lack of bulk directly results in constipation (slower transit time in the intestine that in extreme cases may be up to two weeks), and smaller, harder faeces. In the colon this may contribute to a disease called diverticular disease, where the increased pressure required to propel the contents may cause small hernias called diverticula (diverticulosis). When these become inflamed the disease called diverticulitis develops. Appendicitis is a somewhat similar condition. Dietary fibre, on the other hand, absorbs water and results in larger, softer contents which require less pressure to be moved.

Increased abdominal straining on passing faeces also has been implicated in a number of conditions such as hiatus hernia, varicose veins (fed by major abdominal veins) and even piles (haemorrhoids). At least one component of dietary fibre namely guar gum, reduces the rate of absorption of certain nutrients, notably glucose. This may prevent the onset or ameliorate the effect of diabetes which has been associated with low-fibre high-energy diets. There may be an inadequate clearing of cholesterol and associated substances, leading to a buildup and a tendency to precipitate in the blood vessels thus causing plaque formation and cardiovascular problems, or in the gall bladder causing gallstones.

As stated above, in the West, three times more fat and three times less fibre on average is consumed than in the Third World. Certain emulsifying agents (bile salts) are secreted by the liver, in bile, in response to this increased fat in the diet. These may be broken down by bacteria in the colon and may produce cancer-risk substances. In the presence of fibre, however, these substances can be mopped-up and eliminated rapidly. Unfortunately, diets which are higher in fat are generally lower in dietary fibre, so the risk of colon cancer is increased. Several of the abovementioned conditions if not treated are potentially fatal.

Table 12.1. Dietary Fibre Compendium

FOOD GROUP	DIETARY FIBRE
Milk and products	Nil
Eggs	Nil
Meat and fish	Nil
Fats and oils	Nil
Grain and products	Very high, variable
Nuts and pulses	Very high, variable
Root vegetables	Medium, variable
Leaf vegetables	Low, variable
Fruit	Medium, variable
Sweets	Nil

13

Lipids

Common Name

Lipids.

Alternative Names

Fats. Oils. Neutral Fat.
Triglycerides (or Triacylglycerols).
Fatty Acids (saturated, mono- and poly- unsaturated).
Saponifiable and non-saponifiable fat.
Lecithin and other phospholipids.
Cholesterol and derivatives.
Ketones or Ketone Bodies.
(Alcohol).

Some of the above are specific compounds.

Nature

Lipids are a diverse mixture of substances, originally defined as compounds which dissolve in organic solvents (fat solvents) but not in water. This is still a good definition. Lipids include all traditional fats and oils as well as a wide range of substances and derivatives found in close association with them in nature. Dietary lipids may be classified under the following headings:

- Simple lipids, such as fats and oils, containing chiefly the neutral fats called triacylglycerols (triglycerides).

- Compounds such as the phospholipids, for example lecithin, known chemically as the phosphatidyl- cholines and inositols.

- Derived lipids such as glycerol, the free fatty acids, the ketone bodies and the sterols such as cholesterol.

The body can synthesise all types of lipids from other components in the diet, except certain polyunsaturated fatty acids. Like carbohydrates, it is not relevant therefore to list the sources of each type of lipid. The total lipid in the diet is more relevant from the nutritional point of view than the individual components. However, there is an increasing awareness that there should be less of the saturated and more of the unsaturated type of fatty acids in the diet (see the following chapter on the fatty acids). Apart from the few essential fatty acids (Chapter 15), there is no absolute minimum requirement for lipid in general. However, if the total energy intake is dramatically decreased body proteins are eventually broken down. This results in a negative nitrogen balance as explained in Chapter 16 which deals with the proteins. One way of off-setting this effect is to eat a large amount of protein and carbohydrate. Too much protein in the diet has its own disadvantages however, and one has to eat two or three times as much carbohydrate or protein to make up for every gram of lipid lacking in the diet. By far the simplest way to keep the levels in proportion is to eat a reasonable amount of lipid. By doing this, it is assured that the minimum amount of essential fatty acids is obtained. Also, the phospholipids in fatty foods contain choline and inositol (which is recommended by some authors). Also, various lipids contain the fat-soluble vitamins A, D, E and K, which are lacking elsewhere. Cholesterol, although not essential, also needs to be considered. This is because it is advisable to limit the intake of cholesterol to reasonable levels because in excess it may become harmful.

Biological Functions

- Lipids are universally distributed in the body and make up several key structural components in all cells. The total lipid stored in the body is very variable. The percentage lipid in various people of different body types is compared in Table 13.1. The total lipid stored in the body of the standard man is equivalent to 400,000 kJ (or about 35 days' supply). On the other hand, the standard woman stores the equivalent of 600,000 kJ (which could last her around 60 days).

- The human body is ideally adapted to store fat. Special cells called adipocytes make up the adipose tissue which is widely distributed particularly under the skin. This is a well organised tissue and is principally involved with the production and storage of the triacylglycerol variety of lipid. Each of these lipids consists of a short section called glycerol onto which are attached three fatty acids. Olive oil and margarine are examples of plant origin and butter is an example of animal origin.

- Lipid is the most efficient long-term store of body energy and is quickly mobilised when needed.

- Lipids add palatability, flavour and aroma, to food and remain longer in the stomach than other food-stuffs thus delays the return of hunger.

- A mixed lipid intake, in addition, ensures an adequate supply of essential fatty acids and fat-soluble vitamins which are essential to health.

- Polyunsaturated fatty acid derivatives include the prostaglandin hormones.

- Cholesterol derivatives include all the steroid hormones and vitamin D.

- The full utilisation of lipid depends on carbohydrate intermediates.

- Lipid spares protein breakdown.

Requirement

There is no recommended daily intake of lipid except for infants, but certain factors put the acceptable adult intake around 20 to 35 g per day. Generally, daily intakes are considerably in excess of this value. The best sources of lipids include oils, butter, nuts, pâté, bacon, some cheeses, duck, chocolates, cakes and sausages. A lipid compendium is included for information (Table 13.2).

Toxicity

Excessive intake of certain lipids may result in vitamin toxicities. Vitamins A and D in particular are found in high concentrations in certain fats and oils. Lipids themselves are non-toxic. However, excessive and prolonged intake (particularly in conjunction with low dietary fibre intake) has been associated with the development of certain types of cancer, for example cancer of the colon. A high energy intake may ultimately lead to obesity and associated problems. In some cases of obesity fat may outweigh all the other material in the body!

Deficiency

A lack of lipid intake results in a concomitant lack of all associated nutrients, such as the fat-soluble vitamins, each of which has its own deficiency signs. Similarly, a lack of essential fatty acids may lead to vision problems. Prolonged lipid deficiency can result in a loss of weight and a negative nitrogen balance.

Table 13.1. Body lipid content (as a percentage of total weight)

Body type	Male	Female
Thin	5 - 9	15 - 19
Average	10 - 14	20 - 24
Plump	15 - 19	25 - 29
Fat	20 - 24	30 - 34
Obese	25, plus	35, plus

Table 13.2. Lipid Compendium

FOOD GROUP	LIPID LEVEL
Milk and products	Medium
Eggs	Medium
Meat and fish	Medium, variable
Fats and oils	Very high
Grain and products	Very low
Nuts / Pulses	Very high / Nil
Root vegetables	Nil
Leaf vegetables	Nil
Fruit	Nil
Sweets	Nil

14

Fatty Acids (and Cholesterol)

In the previous chapter the lipids in general were considered. The main purpose of this separate chapter is to consider some of the differences between the three types of fatty acids. With just two exceptions (which will be considered in the following chapter), the fatty acids are not essential nutrients. Nevertheless, they deserve special attention.

Fatty Acids

Fatty acids are derived lipids of great variety, and about 100 different acids have so far been isolated from various foods. They are all defined chemically as aliphatic (usually long-chain) monocarboxylic acids and fall into three broad classes depending on the number of double bonds they contain. Saturated acids contain no double bonds. Monounsaturated (monoenoic) acids, as the name suggests, contain one double bond. And, polyunsaturated (polyenoic) acids contain more than one double bond.

In addition, there are a large number of relatively unusual derivatives which are of no nutritional significance except for the fact that they may produce toxic effects in high concentrations. Castor oil for example contains ricinoleic acid which is a good purgative in small doses. This is classified as a therapeutic not a nutritive effect. A number of seed oils contain a cyclopropene acid, which in the case of cottonseed oil must be removed before the oil can be used to make margarine. Many oils contain traces of other adulterants, such as the terpene gossypol, which is highly toxic and inhibits several dehydrogenase enzymes. Indeed, it could be argued that cholesterol itself is a natural adulterant associated with many animal fats.

The most obvious lipids in the diet are visible meat fats and renderings and the vegetable oils. But lipids occur universally and, in trace amounts, they are an integral component of all cells. Lipid predominantly occurs as triacylglycerols (triglycerides) where each molecule contains three (often different) fatty acids joined to glycerol. For simplicity, it may be assumed that 95 percent of the total lipid in the diet is in the form of triacylglycerols and that fatty acids themselves make up 95 percent of these molecules (the remaining 5 percent being glycerol). In other words, approximately 90 percent of the total lipid in the diet is composed of fatty acids.

The lipid content of various food groups is indicated in a compendium (Table 14.1). The average total lipid content in different food groups varies from 0 to 100 percent, but there is considerable variation even within each food group. Because of this variation, it is pointless to lump various values together to construct a percentage distribution table for each group. The distribution in different food items, however, is of great nutritional interest. The most concentrated sources are pure fats and oils, nuts, cream and some cheeses.

For practical purposes, food containing less that 1 percent lipid is classified as having no fat. This does not mean that the value is actually zero. All fruit and vegetables for example contain fatty acids at levels in the range 0.1 to 1.0 grams per 100 grams, and these have a high proportion of polyunsaturated fatty acids. However, one would have to eat 1 kilogram of lettuce to obtain just 2 grams of fat (so the values are negligible). Apart from pure fats and nuts, significant lipid is obtained from the dairy products, milk, cheese and eggs, and in the meat, oily fish and poultry group.

It should be stressed that it is not possible to separate the intake of different fatty acids in a particular food item. For example, just two eggs (about 100 grams), will provide about 1.3 grams of polyunsaturated, about 5 grams of monounsaturated and about 4 grams of saturated fatty acids, not to mention 0.5 grams of cholesterol, all at the same time. The same considerations apply to all food items. It is the average daily balance of the three types of acid, and not so much their total value or the value in each food item, which really counts.

It has been recommended to reduce our overall consumption of saturated fats while at the same time increasing our overall consumption of monounsaturated and polyunsaturated fats. The ultimate goal should be as follows: one third of the total lipid intake in each of the three fatty acid forms, and preferable not more than one third of our total energy intake as lipid (nominally 30 percent, with 10 percent contributed by each type of fatty acid). But as explained above, there is no simple way of guaranteeing this balance.

A general reduction of about 25 percent fat (for people on the average Western diet), and a switch from some saturated to polyunsaturated sources would be a step in the right direction. As a first approximation, a switch from animal to vegetable fats is a simple rule to follow. There are many exceptions however, and the shopping list in Table 14.2, gives a more detailed summary. As a matter of interest, the nutritionally dominant fatty acids, as presently eaten in a typical Western diet, are listed in Table 14.3. Some further details on individual fatty acids are given in Appendix A2.

Although a great variety of different fatty acids occur in nature (see Appendix A2), unlike the essential amino acids each of which has a distinct nutritional requirement, individual fatty acids, with one or two notable exceptions, are not nutritionally essential as they are metabolically interconvertible in the body. The average ratio of *cis*- to *trans*- monounsaturated fatty acids in the diet is approximately 6:1. A number of *trans*- forms of polyunsaturated fatty acids also occur in the diet.

The chain length of fatty acids occurring in the diet can have any value up to 30 carbon atoms or more, but are principally even numbered, with values from about 14 to 24 carbon atoms being the most common. Lower values occur in milk products, whereas higher values tend to occur in certain fish oils and waxes. The most common saturated fatty acids have from 4 to 24 carbon atoms with chain lengths from 14 to 18 carbon atoms predominating. The most common monounsaturated fatty acids have from 14 to 22 carbon atoms. And the most common polyunsaturated fatty acids have from 16 to 24 carbon atoms, and may have from two to six double bonds.

The most common polyunsaturated fatty acid is linoleic with 18 carbons and two double bonds, both in the *cis-* conformation (which means that the groups are on opposite sides of the double bond). The most common monounsaturated fatty acids are oleic and palmitoleic with 18 and 16 carbons respectively, and one *cis-* double bond. And, the most common saturated fatty acids are stearic and palmitic, also with 18 and 16 carbons but with no double bonds. In fact, any chain length from 2 carbons to 22 carbons can occur (usually with an even number of carbons). Acetic acid has 2 carbons and occurs in vinegar. Butyric acid has 4 carbons and occurs in butter. Even the 1 carbon formic acid occurs in nature (in nettles and ant stings) but not as a food acid. Higher fatty acids, such as those found in certain waxes and cutins, (sometimes with up to 30 carbons, or more), are extremely rare in animals, because they do not melt at body temperature and hence cannot be metabolised properly in the body.

In this connection it is worth noting that all fat appears hard or solid on a piece of cold meat, but in the living body it is in a liquid or semi-liquid state. On the other hand, in certain fish, their low melting oils protect them from freeing up in arctic seas. As a general rule, the longer the carbon chain the higher the melting point. Secondly, polyunsaturated chains generally have a lower melting point than corresponding saturated ones of the same chain length. Oils are simply fats that are liquid at room temperature.

Fatty acids are relatively non-toxic, but there are dangers associated with eating too much fatty acids, and in particular polyunsaturated ones. In addition to the three main types of fatty acids considered above, there are a number of derivatives which occur widely in nature in minute amounts. These include branched chains, oxy groups (keto, hydroxy and epoxy), aldehydes and higher alcohols, *trans-* double bonds, triple bonds and cyclic groups. Fatty acids at experimentally high levels affect enzymes. An excess causes inhibition due to binding. Erucic acid, a long-chain monounsaturated acid found in rape-seed oil, can produce toxic effects in animals such as fatty deposits in heart tissue. The naturally occurring *cis-* acids have their main groups on opposite sides of the double bonds but *trans-* acids exist which have their main groups on the same side of the double bond causing kinks in the molecule. The *trans-* acids are mainly synthetic in origin although some do occur naturally. These also occur during the hardening of oils for the manufacture of margarine. They appear to be relatively harmless but research is continuing. High concentrations of cyclopropene fatty acids, such as sterculic acid, alter the permeability of membranes causing leakage. It seems that they inhibit the natural conversion of stearic to oleic acid in some way. These acids occur as adulterants in some vegetable oils. Very low levels seem to be harmless, but high doses have proved fatal in animals. Such acids contain a triangular carbon bridge across an otherwise normal single or double bond. Finally, oxidation of unsaturated fatty acids may give rise to toxic peroxides which can react adversely with enzymes and even nucleic acids. This oxidation in part helps to explain the toxic effect of high pressure oxygen as previously mentioned in Chapter 5. In nature, unsaturated acids are accompanied by natural antioxidants such as vitamin E. This is not always true of food preparations.

Research is ongoing with regard to the effects of fatty acids on cholesterol levels. Briefly, the facts appear to be as follows:

- Polyunsaturated fatty acids tend to reduce blood cholesterol levels

- Monounsaturated fatty acids also tend to reduce blood cholesterol levels

- Saturated fatty acids tend to increase blood cholesterol levels

- Cholesterol itself also tends to increase blood cholesterol levels.

Increased levels of cholesterol in the blood have been associated with the formation of plaque in the arteries (atherosclerosis). The formation of plaque is associated with a range of cardio-vascular disorders.

So the current debate hinges on three questions, namely:

- Whether cholesterol is an active agent in plaque formation or not
- Whether a reduction in blood cholesterol should be the primary goal in preventing arteriosclerosis in the first place
- Whether plaque is reversible or irreversible, once formed.

In the meantime, research continues to find dietary modifications that can ultimately prevent (even reverse) plaque formation. Associated with the polyunsaturated fatty acids, in particular, are the essential fatty acids which are considered in the following chapter.

Cholesterol

Cholesterol itself is a member of the steroid or sterol group of chemicals which contain the four fused rings known as the cyclopentanoperhydrophenanthrene nucleus. The chemical name for cholesterol is 3-hydroxy-5,6-cholestene. Cholesterol was found in gallstones in the 18th century. During the 19th century, Chevreul, Bertelot and others began to isolate it in pure form and characterise its chemical properties. Unlike the fatty acids which may form salts or soaps with alkali (a process called saponification), cholesterol does not form salts, in other words it is non-saponifiable. There is a large amount of cholesterol in the brain and other nervous tissues. The liver, which is the site of synthesis of cholesterol, is also a good source. Cholesterol is a component of the blood where about two-thirds of it is linked mainly to polyunsaturated fatty acids. Much of the cholesterol is carried on specific proteins in the blood called lipoproteins. Cholesterol also occurs in the skin and many other tissues. The steroid hormones, vitamin D, and the bile salts are all derivatives of the basic cholesterol structure.

Cholesterol is synthesised in the body and, therefore, is not essential but is liable to individual metabolic variation. On average, about 1 gram is synthesised per day by the normal adult. Cholesterol occurs in food and this source can increase or supplement the natural amounts produced in the body. The best sources of cholesterol include kidneys, liver, meat fat, eggs, butter, prawns, crabs and lobster. But dietary cholesterol is not essential and some authors would even argue the opposite. Current intake in the West nay be as high as 500 milligrams per day. The preferred daily intake should be 300 milligrams, or less. Blood cholesterol tends to rise with age. A satisfactory level of cholesterol in the blood would be around 120 mg per 100 ml blood, or less. As concentrations increase over this level, there is a gradual increase in the risk of coronary heart disease. At a level twice the average, that is 240 mg per 100 ml, the risk of death is 35 percent greater. And at levels over three times the population average, that is 360 mg per 100 ml, the risk of death has doubled. Virtually all the cholesterol in the diet comes from animal sources, as the cholesterol compendium illustrates (Table 14.4). In recent years the emphasis has switched away from reducing cholesterol intake itself to reducing saturated fatty acid intake and increasing polyunsaturated fatty acid intake.

Table 14.1. Total Lipid compendium

FOOD GROUP	CHOLESTEROL
Milk / Products	Low, variable / Medium
Eggs	Low
Meat and fish	Medium, variable
Fats and Oils	Very High
Grain and products	Very low
Nuts / Pulses	High / Low
Root vegetables	Nil
Leaf vegetables	Nil
Fruit	Nil
Sweets	Nil

Table 14.2. Comparative lists of unsaturated versus saturated fat sources

FOOD GROUP	Sources relatively rich in unsaturated fatty acids	Sources relatively rich in saturated fatty acids
Milk and products	----	Milk, Cream Most cheeses Butter
Eggs	Egg yolks	Egg yolks
Meat and fish	Fish, especially oily fish. Shellfish Salmon, Sardines	Animal fat products Most meats (Pork, Lamb, Beef, Turkey with fat)
Fats and oils	Most vegetable oils (Olive oil, Safflower, Soya bean, Sunflower and Corn oils	Coconut and Palm kernel oil
Grain and products	Flax seeds	Trace
Nuts	Most nuts (Hazelnuts, Peanuts, Walnuts, Almonds, Pecans, Brazil nuts)	Coconuts Palm kernel oil
Pulses	Beans Peas	----
Fruit and vegetables	Avocados Strawberries Berries Leafy greens, Broccoli, Squash, Melon, Mango	Trace
Sweets	----	----

Table 14.3. Nutritionally important fatty acids (intakes expressed as a percentage of total fatty acid intake)

FATTY ACID	Typical relative intake	Number of carbon atoms
SATURATED		
Palmitic acid	24	16
Stearic acid	11	18
Myristic acid	7	14
Lauric acid	2	12
All others	5	---
MONOUNSATURATED		
Oleic acid	32	18
Palmitoleic acid	3	16
All others	4	---
POLYUNSATURATED		
Linoleic acid	9	18
α-Linolenic acid	2	18
All others	1	---

Table 14.4. Cholesterol Compendium

FOOD GROUP	CHOLESTEROL
Milk and products	Medium, variable
Eggs	Very high
Meat and fish	Medium, variable
Fats / Oils	High / Very low
Grain and products	Nil
Nuts and pulses	Nil
Root vegetables	Nil
Leaf vegetables	Nil
Fruit	Nil
Sweets	Nil

15

Essential Fatty Acids: Linoleic Acid and α-Linolenic Acid

Common Name

Essential Fatty Acids (EFA).

Alternative Names
Linoleic acid. Linolenic acid; α- or γ- forms.
GLA. DGLA, dihomo-γ-Linolenic acid.
Arachidonic acid.
Timnodonic (or eicosapentaenoic) acid.
Stearidonic acid.
Polyunsaturated fatty acids (PUFA).
ω-3, ω-6 Acids
(n-6, n-9)-Acids. delta-5,8,11,14-Tetraenoic acids.
(Prostaglandins).
Vitamin F.

Some of the above include specific compounds, series or derivatives.

Nature

The essential fatty acids were discovered following an observation by Evans and Burr in 1928. The two primary essential fatty acids are linoleic acid and α-linolenic acid. All the other so-called essential metabolites can be synthesised in the body provided these two starting materials are provided in the diet. Regrettably, these fatty acids have names that differ in different books. The first table (Table 15.1) in this chapter is therefore a simple synonym list to make cross references easier. The first names in the list will be used throughout the remainder of the chapter. Only fatty acids which give rise to biologically active prostaglandins are defined as having essential fatty acid activity. Many intermediates and synthetic compounds are now known to have such activity. Research using such compounds has discovered that there are three main series of prostaglandin. Prostaglandins are derivatives of polyunsaturated acids of the essential type, which like hormones have profound biochemical, pharmacological and physiological effects in the body, and yet are completely natural compounds.

In plants, oleic acid can be converted into linoleic acid which in turn is converted into α-linolenic acid. In animals, on the other hand, oleic acid cannot be converted into linoleic acid, but linoleic acid in the diet can be converted into γ-linolenic acid and thence into dihomo-γ-linolenic acid and arachidonic acid. Plants cannot convert linoleic acid into γ-linolenic acid and animals cannot convert linoleic acid to α-linolenic acid. The only difference between α- and γ-linolenic acid is in the position of one double bond in the carbon chain.

All fatty acids with essential fatty acid activity give rise to prostaglandins in the body. An interesting structural feature which is common to many of the active fatty acids is the occurrence of double bonds in the n-6 and n-9 positions from the omega end. Interestingly linoleic, linolenic, dihomo-γ-linolenic and arachidonic acids all have this same feature in common. It is now believed the any fatty acid capable of being converted to a C19:4, C20:4 or C21:4 acid with the key double bond structure (5,8,11,14) from the carboxyl end, will have essential fatty acid activity and be capable of forming an active prostaglandin in the body. See Appendix A2 for details of the structural and omega codes.

Considerable structural variation is possible with unsaturated fatty acids. Double bonds may be introduced at various points along the carbon chain and up to six double bonds are found in certain acids. However, the most common number of double bonds are 3, 4 and 5 respectively, as exemplified by the three key prostaglandin precursors. The key to whether a particular acid has essential fatty acid activity or not depends on the way it is metabolised in the body.

A series of enzymes called delta (Δ) desaturases are able to insert double bonds into various sites on saturated fatty acid chains. Two key enzymes namely, Δ9-desaturase and Δ6-desaturase, insert double bonds at carbon positions 9 and 6 from the carboxyl end, respectively. Double bonds cannot be inserted between the first double bond and the carboxyl group. However, fatty acids can be elongated by addition of two-carbon units, and further double bonds can then be inserted. In this way, depending on the starting material, a range of different unsaturated acids may be produced in the body, but only some of these are biologically active (Figure 15.1).

Unsaturated fatty acids may be named according to the number and positions of their double bonds. For example, *n*-6 acids have a double bond between carbon 6 and 7 counting from the carboxyl end of the molecule. Further examples are given in Appendix A2. Most if not all fatty acids with the *n*-6 structure have essential fatty acid activity. Linoleic and arachidonic acid are *n*-6 fatty acids. α-Linolenic acid also has some essential fatty acid activity. This acid is a *n*-3 fatty acid. On the other hand, oleic acid (*n*-9) and palmitoleic acid (*n*-7), have no essential fatty acid activity. Table 15.1. lists synonyms of some essential fatty acids and metabolites.

Figure 15.1. Metabolic pathways arising from the primary essential
fatty acids, linoleic and α-linolenic acids.

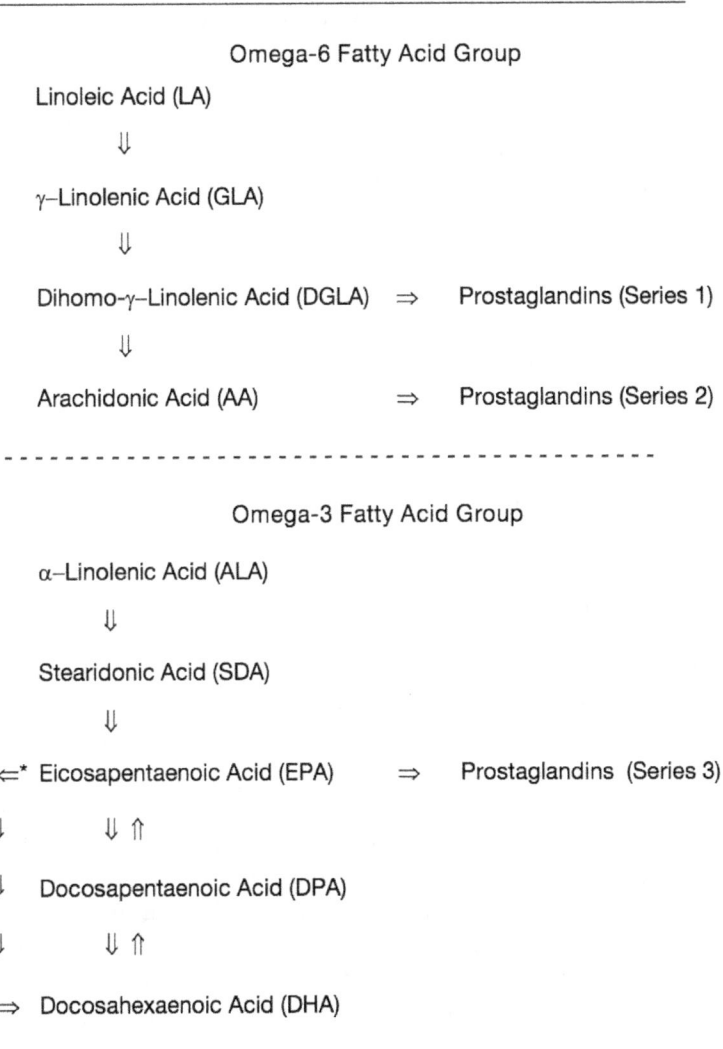

Omega-6 Fatty Acid Group

Linoleic Acid (LA)

⇓

γ–Linolenic Acid (GLA)

⇓

Dihomo-γ–Linolenic Acid (DGLA)　⇒　　Prostaglandins (Series 1)

⇓

Arachidonic Acid (AA)　　　　　　⇒　　Prostaglandins (Series 2)

- -

Omega-3 Fatty Acid Group

α–Linolenic Acid (ALA)

⇓

Stearidonic Acid (SDA)

⇓

⇐* Eicosapentaenoic Acid (EPA)　　⇒　　Prostaglandins (Series 3)

⇓　　　⇓ ⇑

⇓　　Docosapentaenoic Acid (DPA)

⇓　　　⇓ ⇑

⇒　Docosahexaenoic Acid (DHA)

* The pathway from EPA to DHA is called the Sprechner shunt.

The most common essential fatty acids in food are linoleic and α-linolenic acid. In general, with a few exceptions, only traces of the other intermediates are found. This relative lack of intermediates in food is nutritionally unimportant as they are all produced by enzymes in the body. The main exceptions are certain fish which contain significant amounts of eicosapentaenoic acid (EPA), and organ meat which is generally rich in arachidonic acid. The prostaglandins as such do not occur, because they are present only in infinitesimal amounts in living cells, and are rapidly broken down as well.

Nutritional information on the essential fatty acids is far from complete and still remains the subject of intensive investigations. It has recently been suggested that another polyunsaturated fatty acid with six double bonds called docosahexaenoic acid may be essential in certain circumstances. This acid is abundant in fish oils and many phospholipids.

The key enzyme controlling the final step in prostaglandin formation in animals is prostaglandin synthase. Two further series of compounds which are very closely related to the prostaglandins are the thromboxanes and the prostacyclins. Thromboxanes are synthesised by the platelets in the blood and prostacyclins occur in endothelial cells, which line the walls of arteries and veins. The chief function of the thromboxanes (together with a host of other factors) is to encourage blood to clot. The prostacyclins counteract this effect in the walls of the blood vessels where clotting could result in strokes due to thrombosis. The prostacyclins also help to prevent the deposits of plaque which clog up the arteries and leads to high blood pressure and heart disease. The natural balance between the thromboxanes and the prostacyclins is a very delicate one. Prostaglandins, thromboxanes and prostacyclins together are termed prostanoids. Prostanoids together with the leukotrienes all contain 20 carbon atoms and are termed eicosanoids. Leukotrienes are inflammatory mediators produced in leukocytes by the oxidation of arachidonic acid and eicosapentaenoic acid by the enzyme arachidonate 5-lipoxygenase.

There are three main families of prostaglandins namely, series 1, 2 and 3, respectively. Series 1 is synthesised only from dihomo-γ-linolenic acid. Series 2 is synthesised only from arachidonic acid. Both of these series therefore arise from linoleic acid. On the other hand, series 3 arises only from eicosapentaenoic acid, which is a metabolite of α-linolenic acid. It is theoretically possible therefore to alter the balance of these prostaglandin series in the body by adjusting the amounts of linoleic and α-linolenic acid in the diet. Fish is a rich source of eicosapentaenoic acid itself, and at the same time is poor in dihomo-γ-linolenic and arachidonic acid. Eskimos who live on fish essentially, therefore, have substituted the series-3 precursor for a series-2 or series-1 precursor. An interesting feature of this substitution is that while the prostacyclins thus produced are biologically active, the corresponding thromboxanes are not. It has been observed that Eskimos have very little heart disease but they do have a tendency to bleed. Autopsies reveal that they have little or no clogging up of their arteries despite having an excessive intake of fat in their diet. This is just one other piece of evidence supporting the view that it is not so much the total fat intake which is important, but the balance of the type of fatty acids eaten which determines the overall benefit to health.

Biological Functions

- Essential fatty acids are precursors to several bioactive mediators, such as prostaglandins, thromboxanes, prostacyclins and leukotrienes.

- Linoleic acid, arachidonic acid and docosahexaenoic acid, are the most common polyunsaturated fatty acids found in tissues.

- Linoleic and α-linolenic acid and their immediate metabolites are not themselves biologically active.

- Like hormones, prostaglandins have profound biochemical, pharmacological and physiological effects in the body, and yet are completely natural compounds.

- The essential fatty acids are widely distributed and form the structural lipids, particularly the phospholipids, in the cell membranes. The integrity of cell membranes is particularly important in nerve cells, for example, infants have a clear need for the essential fatty acids for brain development (and for growth).

- Derivatives of the prostaglandins, namely the thromboxanes and the prostacyclins, regulate the mechanism of blood clotting.

- The essential fatty acids regulate many aspects of metabolism particularly the metabolism of lipids.

- Both ω-6 and ω-3 fatty acids are important structural components of cell membranes.

- The phospholipids of the brain contain high proportions of docosahexaenoic acid and arachidonic acid, suggesting they are important to the central nervous system.

- Docosahexaenoic acid is important for visual and neurological development. Docosahexaenoic acid is found in high concentrations in the retina of the eye.

- Dihomo-γ-linolenic acid is found in large quantities in cartilage.

- Dihomo-γ-linolenic acid has been found to decrease osteoblastic activity

- Fish oil consumption, may decrease the risk of coronary heart disease.

- Long-chain ω-3 polyunsaturated fatty acids can exert anti-inflammatory effects. Fish oil supplementation may reduce the requirement for anti-inflammatory medication in certain patients.

- Increasing eicosapentaenoic and docosahexaenoic acid intake may be beneficial in certain individuals with type 2 diabetes, especially those with elevated serum triglycerides.

- High (pharmacological) doses of essential fatty acids, particularly ω-3, may help to alleviate certain types of depression.

Requirement

Linoleic acid, an ω-6 fatty acid, and α-linolenic acid, an ω-3 fatty acid, are essential fatty acids because they cannot be synthesized by humans. The long-chain ω-3 fatty acids, eicosapentaenoic acid and docosahexaenoic acid, can be synthesized in the body from α-linolenic acid, but due to low conversion efficiency (particularly in males), they may be considered as conditionally essential nutrients and it is recommended to obtain them from additional sources. It has been suggested that a minimum of 1 to 2 percent of the total energy requirement should be supplied in the form of linoleic acid. This level is sufficient to prevent deficiency states. It is considered that an intake of around 20 grams of linoleic acid per day for males and 10 for females should meet adult requirements. It has been estimated that the average Western diet supplies 20 to 25 grams of linoleic acid per day so a deficiency is extremely unlikely, except after a prolonged fat-free diet.

It has also been suggested that a minimum of 0.5 percent of the total energy requirement should be supplied in the form of α-linolenic acid. An intake of around 2 grams of α-linolenic acid per day for males and around 1 gram for females should meet adult requirements. No daily minimum has been set for docosahexaenoic acid.

The best sources are foods rich in other polyunsaturated fatty acids (see previous chapter). The sparse occurrence of key intermediates (pre-formed) in food is shown for interest in Table 15.2.

Toxicity

The essential fatty acid levels found in food are non-toxic. Excessive intakes would first result in nausea due to over-ingestion of the accompanying lipids. High doses of essential fatty acids may increase blood clotting time. Prolonged excessive intakes would have the same results as for other lipids. High (experimental) concentrations of some pure compounds are likely to cause metabolic disturbances.

Deficiency

Under normal circumstances a deficiency is impossible. Infants and orphanage children have been known to develop deficiencies which are corrected on administering linoleic acid. Patients on prolonged intravenous feeding may also develop symptoms. Essential fatty acid deficiency can result in impaired brain function, particularly in the young. Another clinical sign is dermatitis, a scaly skin condition, characterised by dryness and water permeability due to lack of natural waxes (sebum).

There may be a decrease in weight, or a cessation of growth in children. Certain metabolic changes may subsequently develop including changes in the fatty acid composition of most tissues accompanied by possible liver and kidney damage. There may be an accumulation of cholesterol. Disturbances in the reproductive system have also been observed in some animals. A disease called sprue which results in an impaired ability to absorb carbohydrates and lipids may indirectly give rise to an essential fatty acid deficiency.

The long-chain omega-3 fatty acids, eicosapentaenoic acid (EPA) and docosahexaenoic acid (DHA), can be synthesized from α-linolenic acid (ALA), but due to low conversion efficiency (particularly in males), it is recommended to obtain EPA and DHA from additional sources. About one tenth of the dietary omega-3 acids are in these forms.

The enzyme prostaglandin synthase is sensitive to a number of drugs including aspirin, which cause inhibition of its activity. In the presence of such drugs the synthesis of certain prostaglandins is depressed and in effect this leads to a temporary deficiency. It has been argued that certain conditions, including individual variation, may result in a general inadequacy of the synthetic pathways involved in essential fatty acid metabolism, even in the absence of drugs. High concentrations of *trans-* unsaturated fatty acids may aggravate essential fatty acid deficiencies possibly by inhibiting desaturase enzymes which help the interconversion of certain precursors.

Table 15.1. Synonyms of the essential fatty acids and some metabolites.

Common Name	Alternative Names	Number of Carbon Atoms	Number of Double Bonds
PRIMARY ESSENTIAL FATTY ACIDS (EFA)			
Linoleic Acid (LA)	*cis-cis*-Linoleic acid all-*cis*-Octadecadienoic acid delta-9,12-Octadecadienoic acid	18	2
α–Linolenic Acid (ALA)	all-*cis*-Octadecatrienoic acid delta-9,12,15-Octadecatrienoic acid	18	3
SOME INTERMEDIATES			
γ–Linolenic Acid (GLA)	all-*cis*-Octadecatrienoic acid delta-6,9,12-Octadecatrienoic acid	18	3
Stearidonic Acid (SDA)	Moroctic acid (all-*cis*) all-*cis*-6,9,12,15-Octadecatetraenoic acid	18	4
KEY PROSTAGLANDIN PRECURSORS			
Prostaglandin series 1			
Dihomo-γ–Linolenic acid (DGLA),	Eicosatrienoic acid (all-*cis*) *all-cis*-8,11,14-Eicosatrienoic acid Mead acid	20	3
Prostaglandin series 2			
Arachidonic acid (AA)	Eicosatetraenoic acid, (all-*cis*) delta-5,8,11,14-Eicosatetraenoic acid	20	4
Prostaglandin series 3			
Eicosapentaenoic acid (EPA)	Timnodonic acid (all-*cis*) delta-5,8,11,14,17-Eicosapentaenoic acid	20	5
RECENTLY POSTULATED AS ESSENTIAL			
Docosahexaenoic acid (DHA)	all-*cis*-4,7,10,13,16,19-Docosahexaenoic acid delta-4,7,10,13,16,19-Docosahexaenoic acid	22	6

Eicosa is a term which implies 20 carbon atoms and may also be spelt icosa.

Docosa is a term which implies 22 carbon atoms.

Most of the natural unsaturated fatty acids are in the all-*cis* configuration.

Table 15.2. Some levels of immediate prostaglandin precursors in food
(all values given as a percentage of the total fatty acid content)

FOOD	Dihomo-γ-linolenic acid (Series 1)	Arachidonic acid (Series 2)	Eicosapentaenoic acid (Series 3)
Shellfish	----	3	19
Fish, various	----	3 or less	14 or less
Chicken	trace	6 - 3	2 - 1
Turkey	----	5	2
Kidneys, various	trace	11 - 7	----
Liver, various	trace	14 - 7	----
Beef	----	1	----
Other meats	----	trace	trace
Corn	----	3	3
Soya beans	----	----	trace

Many values are nil, or unknown. Only traces are found in most foods.

The eicosapentaenoic acid values include traces of stearidonic acid, if present.

16
PROTEINS (AND NUCLEIC ACIDS)

Common Name

Proteins.

Alternative Names

Polypeptides.
Amino Acids.
Dietary Nitrogen.

Nature

The word protein from the Greek *proteios*, meaning holding first place, was coined by Berzelius in 1838. Proteins are in many respects simpler though infinitely more varied than carbohydrates or lipids. They are all composed of amino acids which are the chief sources of nitrogen and sulphur in the diet. Proteins, therefore, cannot be fully derived from carbohydrate or lipid. In contrast, carbohydrates can be derived from the glycerol in certain lipids and also from some amino acids. And, lipids can be derived from carbohydrates.

Proteins may be divided into two broad groups, the simple proteins and the conjugated proteins. Simple proteins contain only amino acids and there are many examples as follows. Albumins and globulins are very varied and widely distributed in nature and are easily digested. Most globular proteins are also in this class and when conjugated they give rise to numerous enzymes. Specific plant proteins include the glutelins and prolamines which are rich in proline. The protamines and histones are very rich in arginine and low in cysteine, thus they function as basic proteins often found in association with nucleic acids. Finally, the scleroproteins which are generally fibrous are also widely distributed and contain glycine, alanine and proline in large amounts. They include the structural proteins found in cartilage, skin, bone and hair, such as the collagen and keratin. From the nutritional point of view, it is only the amino acid composition which is important in the diet, not the structure or source of the protein.

There are twenty common amino acids but not all of these occur in each type of protein. A given protein may be rich in some and poor, or even completely deficient, in other amino acids. On the other hand, some proteins have a balanced distribution of all the amino acids, at least, all the essential ones. Proteins from different sources may therefore be nutritionally complete or incomplete, depending on their exact composition. This concept of completeness will be considered again in the next chapter.

The conjugated proteins contain not only amino acids but additional components. These proteins which are subdivided according to the nature of the additional component include a wide range of biologically active molecules. Some typical members of this family include the following: glycoproteins which contain carbohydrates, lipoproteins which contain lipid, nucleoproteins which are conjugated to nucleic acids, metalloproteins which contain metallic minerals, phosphoproteins which contain phosphorous, chromoproteins which contain various pigments and include the important haemoglobin molecule (sometimes distinguished as haemoproteins), flavoproteins which include riboflavin (one of the B complex vitamins), and most enzymes which contain cofactors.

As far as nitrogen balance alone is concerned, it does not matter which amino acids are supplied in the diet, provided a minimum total supply is maintained. However, of the twenty amino acids commonly found in protein, half of them are essential in their own right. The other half are not absolutely essential (although equally important) as they can be interconverted from one to the other in the body as required. One of the key factors determining the requirement for protein is nitrogen balance. The main factors which affect this balance are the growth rate, physical exercise, injury and stress. Typical food intake of nitrogen is 4 – 12 grams per day. The main losses occur in the urine (5 – 10 g), faeces (about 0.6 g), and skin (about 0.2 g) per day. On average, the net gain should equal the net loss in an adult. In children, however, there should be a positive nitrogen balance for growth. Intakes of nitrogen exceeding about 8 grams per day will generally result in a positive nitrogen balance (overall gain of nitrogen), whereas intakes below 8 grams per day will generally result in a negative nitrogen balance (overall loss of nitrogen). As a rough guide, it has been shown that most dietary proteins contain about 16 percent nitrogen. In other words, every 50 g of pure protein will supply about 8 g of nitrogen in the diet. To maintain nitrogen balance, some people would need more than this, and some would need less. In practice, it is not necessary to calculate nitrogen itself in the diet. A correct protein intake ensures that the nitrogen levels are adequately maintained in the body.

Functional Classification

Proteins may be classified functionally according to their role in the body. There are many different functional groups (with considerable overlap), the main ones include the following:

- Catalytic proteins. All enzymes are in this group.

- Digestive proteins. These are the special enzymes found in the alimentary tract.

- Transport proteins. These are found on cell membranes to carry nutrients into the cell.

- Receptor proteins. These also occur on cell membranes to assist the work of the hormones.

- Respiratory proteins. These special enzyme-like proteins convert the energy released from food into a form which can be stored by the cell.

- Defense proteins. These are the antibodies which protect against infection.

- Blood proteins. There are over 100 proteins found in blood with numerous functions. Albumin and globulin are found in the serum and haemoglobin is found in the red blood cells. Some blood proteins act as carriers for the nutrients. These also include the defense proteins and many hormones.

- Hormones. There are many protein-, polypeptide- and amino acid-derived hormones which regulate metabolism and the function of various organs and glands.

- Regulator Proteins. These proteins may activate or repress the function of the genes to produce specific proteins, particularly certain enzymes. As their name suggests, they have a marked regulatory role in the cell.

- Vision proteins. Rhodopsin is the name of the specific vision protein (pigment).

- Contractile proteins. These are highly specialised enzymes involved in muscle contraction. They also have a structural role.

- Ribosomal proteins. These are part of the structure of ribosomes in the cell involved in the synthesis of all proteins.

- Structural proteins. These do not seem to have an active role but they are essential to the structure of the cell and include collagen and keratin.

Biological Functions

- Next to water, protein is the most abundant substance in an average man. In the case of a woman, however, lipid is more plentiful than protein (see Table 3.4) The total protein stored in the body is equivalent to 200,000 kJ in the standard man and about 150,000 kJ in the standard woman. In both cases this amounts to about 17 days' supply.

- Up to twenty different amino acids are used by cells to synthesise various proteins.

- All enzymes are specific proteins, usually combined with an additional cofactor, which are vital for the life of the cell.

- Amino acid fragments serve as the starting material for the synthesis of various nitrogen compounds, particularly the nucleic acids.

- Certain amino acids (glucogenic amino acids) may give rise to carbohydrates, particularly during prolonged low energy intakes.

- Certain amino acids (ketogenic amino acids) may give rise to lipids, also during prolonged low energy intakes.

- Following digestion and absorption, proteins, in particular, give a sensation of warmth called the heat increment of feeding or the thermic effect of food (previously termed the specific dynamic action).

Requirement

The typical adult requirement of protein is around 50 to 60 grams per day of good protein quality which must include all the essential amino acids (see Chapter 28). For adults, the overall requirement is around 0.8 g/kg, so slightly less is required for women. Food sources of protein are indicated in Table 16.1. Foods rich in protein include milk, meat, fish, eggs and beans.

Toxicity

Excessive protein intake tends to elevate temperature and liberate acidic products which appear in the blood and urine. There may be an elevation of blood pressure. As with other energy providing foodstuffs, excessive intake may cause an increase in weight. There may be vomiting, loss of appetite and possible kidney failure in renal patients. There may be a buildup of ammonia particularly in people with poor liver function.

Deficiency

Losses of protein occur as a result of chronic illness, injury or physical stress. Insufficient protein intake results in a loss of weight, tiredness and anaemia. There is a lowered resistance to diseases and toxins, and slower healing, poor concentration and menstruation may become irregular. In children, there is poor growth. Other effects include a generalised decrease in the absorption of nutrients from the gut, fluid imbalance (oedema) and possibly enlargement of the liver with eventual fatty accumulations leading to cirrhosis).

A specific disease called kwashiorkor is common in the Third World, and is essentially due to an inadequate intake of protein, and in particular the essential amino acids. The disease may possibly be complicated if accompanied by a simultaneous energy depletion (protein-calorie deficiency, or marasmus). In extreme cases, there is an accompanying dehydration and loss of salts. The disease can only be corrected by administering an adequate diet of complete protein.

Nucleic Acids

The nucleic acids were first isolated by Meischer in 1869, and termed nucleic acids by Altmann in 1889. However, it was not until 1953 that the full correct structure of DNA was realised by Watson and Crick. The nucleic acids are not essential nutrients. But it has been claimed that under certain circumstances they may become conditionally essential if the rate of synthesis in the body does not match requirements. All nucleic acids are made up of phosphate, carbohydrate and base components, and are often found in association with protein called nucleoprotein. It is the base components which may become rate limiting in certain circumstances. Broadly, the nucleic acids are divided into two principal groups, DNA (deoxyribonucleic acid) and RNA (ribonucleic acid), respectively. The DNA is only found in the nucleus of cells, whereas the RNA is more extensively distributed throughout the cell. The carbohydrate portion is deoxyribose or ribose. Both are simple 5-carbon sugars readily synthesised in the body. These are joined together by phosphate links to form a very long molecule. The bases are also attached, but to a different carbon of the sugar units. One and only one base is attached to each unit, but the entire nucleic acid molecule may consist of thousands or hundreds of thousands of nucleotides. Each nucleotide consists of one sugar, one phosphate and one base unit.

The exact sequence of bases determines the information content of each nucleic acid. There are just four different bases in DNA; two purines called adenine (A), and guanine (G), and two pyrimidines called cytosine (C) and thymine (T). With one exception, the same bases also occur in RNA namely, the purines adenine and guanine, and the pyrimidines cytosine and (instead of thymine), uracil (U). Both purines and pyrimidines are synthesised in the body by enzymes that require several vitamins (particularly some of the B complex) and minerals as cofactors. The vital function of DNA is to contain and propagate the genetic information of the cell. This information is transferred to RNA which in turn transfers it to various proteins in the cell.

Nucleic acid is required for the growth of cells and to regenerate wound tissue and may also promote an increase in memory and mental concentration. Ageing is caused by degeneration or inefficiency of cells. In humans, there is a sequence of six nucleotides, the telomere, which is repeated about 2,500 times at the ends of DNA molecules. These telomeres protect the ends of chromosomes from deterioration. However, some telomeres are lost each time the DNA replicates and the sequence gets shorter. This is associated with one cause of cellular ageing.

It has been claimed that certain cells can be rejuvenated by supplying them with extra nucleic acid. Claims that between 1.0 and 1.5 grams of nucleic acid per day as a supplement can help reduce the effects of ageing are unsubstantiated. Most individuals are able to synthesise all the nucleic acid they need. A deficiency of nucleic acid does not occur in normal individuals at any age.

Foods rich in nucleic acid include yeast, wheat germ, liver, kidney, oily fish, roe, asparagus, mushrooms, onions, spinach, bear and wine. Excessive intake of nucleic acid, however, may aggravate gout in susceptible individuals due to the breakdown of purines to uric acid which may be deposited as crystals. In individuals susceptible to gout it is occasionally necessary to restrict the intake of purines to about half the normal intake, which is 400 mg per day. For this purpose, the following foods should be avoided: liver, kidney, game, anchovies, herrings, sardines, mackerel and scallops. The following foods contain the lowest levels of purines: fruits, most vegetables, nuts, most grains (except whole grain), sweets, fats, oils, eggs and milk.

Table 16.1. Protein compendium

FOOD GROUP	PROTEIN LEVEL
Milk and products	Very high, variable
Eggs	High
Meat and fish	High
Fats and oils	Nil
Grain and products	Medium
Nuts and pulses	Very high
Root vegetables	Very low
Leaf vegetables	Very low
Fruit	Very low
Sweets	Nil

17
AMINO ACIDS

There are perhaps 300 amino acids found in nature. Of these only twenty are used by the cell to elaborate proteins. Of these twenty only half are essential. Of the ten essential amino acids two are better termed conditionally essential. The following Table (17.1) lists the amino acids required to synthesise proteins.

Occasionally additional amino acids are found in proteins, namely hydroxylysine, hydroxyproline and γ–carboxyglutamic acid. These are not used as such in the initial synthesise of proteins but may arise as a result of modification after the protein has been formed. Lysine may be hydroxylated to 5-hydroxylysine, which is found only in collagen and tooth enamel protein. These modifications involve adding a hydroxyl (-OH) group to the existing amino acid. Proline may be hydroxylated to 4-hydroxyproline which also occurs in collagen and in elastin. Traces of 3-hydroxyproline has also been found in collagen only. It should be noted that gelatin is a derivative of collagen produced during cooking. Further consideration of the hydroxy acids is unnecessary as they are both rare and nonessential. Another rare amino acid, namely γ–carboxyglutamic acid, is derived from glutamic acid and may be found in certain vitamin K-dependent clotting factors. Calmodulin is another unique protein containing a trimethylated lysine residue.

Nature

Chemically speaking all the amino acids (except proline) are α-amino acids which have an amino ($-NH_2$) group and a carboxyl (-COOH) group attached to the same carbon called the alpha carbon. The carboxyl group may release its hydrogen and the amino group may take up an additional hydrogen ion (or proton). This results in various ionic forms of amino acids. The ionised carboxyl is negatively charged and the ionic amino group is positively charged. Often the net charge (one negative and one positive) is zero. Such compounds are called zwitterions. This is an important feature of amino acids but need not be further considered at this point.

Another chemical feature of amino acids found in proteins is the fact that they are all L-amino acids. This is a short-hand notation used to denote that the main amino group is on the left when the molecule is represented in the conventional structural formula. (L- is short for the Latin *laevo-* meaning left). D-Amino acids would have the amino group on the right (D- is short for the Latin *dextro-* meaning right). D-Amino acids also occur in nature but they are not used to synthesise proteins and are therefore nutritionally unimportant. The fact that all amino acids except glycine have different groups attached to a particular carbon makes then optically active. (Glycine has two hydrogens attached to the same carbon and is not optically active) This is another property which is not important as far as nutrition is concerned.

Amino acids may be classified in several different ways. The nature of the principle side group attached to the alpha-carbon atom may be used to classify them. There are ten classifications as follows:

- Aliphatic (simple chains which may be either straight or branched)
- Hydroxylic (contain hydroxyl, -OH)
- Sulphur (contain sulphur, -S)
- Carboxylic (containing an extra acidic group, -COOH)
- Amide (containing a substituted carboxyl, -CONH$_2$)
- Amino (containing one or more extra amino groups, – NH$_2$)
- Aromatic (containing a simple six-carbon ring)
- Heterocyclic (containing a simple mixed ring)
- Heterocyclic aromatic (containing different rings which are fused)
- Imino (containing a rarer imino group, –NH–, instead of

the usual amino group)

The ionic character of an amino acid may be specified as acidic, basic or neutral. This is somewhat different from its polar character which may be either polar or polar. Polarity may be conferred by acidic, basic, or some other groups. Table 17.1 lists these and other properties. The ionic and polar character of the various amino acids in a protein determines its overall structural shape and properties.

The metabolic character of an amino acid is probably one of its more important properties as far as nutrition is concerned. Amino acids that give rise to carbohydrate intermediates are termed glucogenic, whereas amino acids that give rise to lipid intermediates are termed ketogenic. Finally, whether an amino acid is nonessential or essential depend on whether the body is capable of synthesising it from other compounds or not. The last column in Table 17.1 lists this characteristic. Two amino acids, histidine and arginine, appear to be essential only for infants during rapid growth, but not for simple maintenance in adults – these are termed conditionally essential amino acids.

Amino acids are involved in a number of general metabolic reactions as well as specific reactions which will be considered in the individual chapters. The general reactions include decarboxylation (removal of the -COOH group) which often gives rise initially to biologically active amines called biogenic amines. These amines are of pharmacological importance in the nervous system. Some products also act as local hormones in various tissues. Another reaction, deamination (removal of the $-NH_2$ group) gives rise to various keto-acids which act as intermediates in carbohydrate or lipid metabolism, hence the designation glucogenic or ketogenic. The removed amino group may either be transferred to another keto-acid to synthesise a new (nonessential) amino acid (transamination), or it can find its way into the urea cycle to form the end-product urea which is eliminated in the urine.

Requirement

Table 17.2 compares the overall protein requirement and the total essential amino acid requirement for adult men and women. The actual amount of essential amino acids required is only a fraction (approximately one-ninth) of the total amino acid (protein) requirement in adults. In the following chapters each of the ten essential amino acids will be considered in detail. The essential amino acid requirement varies less than the total amino acid (protein) requirement throughout life, but the overall protein requirement is considerably lower for infants.

Toxicity

The fact that too much protein could be harmful for infants should not be surprising. The kidney function of infants cannot handle the increased breakdown products of high protein diets.

Excessive protein intake can lead to acidosis, high blood pressure and obesity. A specific toxicity associated with any one amino acid rarely occurs by overeating protein in general. On the other hand, experimental feeding of individual amino acids can produce specific symptoms. Individual amino acids are occasionally used for their therapeutic effects, but toxic effects associated with these regimes are not strictly relevant to the study of nutrition.

Deficiency

For protein synthesis to occur, all the required amino acids must be present at the site of protein synthesis in adequate amounts at the same time. Deficiency of any one of the required amino acids, in particular the essential amino acids, will result in kwashiorkor or, if also accompanied by an energy depletion, marasmus. Briefly, these conditions all result in cessation of grow as the most immediate symptom. This may be complicated in severe chronic cases by wasting of tissues especially muscle, gut disorders, diarrhoea, loss of appetite, weakness and pathology of various glands, including the pancreas, spleen and salivary glands. Other effects include anaemia, oedema of the hands and feet, and low resistance to various infections. The liver becomes enlarged and fatty and there is a decrease in the production of the blood protein, albumin. This results in a fluid imbalance due to disturbances in the oncotic pressure (colloid osmotic pressure) that usually keeps water in the circulatory system. When albumin is decreased, more water is able to enter the tissues resulting in a typical distended abdomen as seen in severely undernourished children. Kwashiorkor is one of the most serious and widespread nutritional problems world-wide.

Table 17.1. Properties the twenty amino acids required to synthesise proteins

Common name	Nature of side group	Ionic character	Polar character	Metabolic character	Human requirement
Glycine	Aliphatic	N	P	G	CE
Alanine	Aliphatic	N	NP	G	NE
Valine	Aliphatic branched	N	NP	G	E
Leucine	Aliphatic branched	N	NP	K	E
Isoleucine	Aliphatic branched	N	NP	G & K	E
Serine	Hydroxylic	N	P	G	CE
Threonine	Hydroxylic	N	P	G	E
Cysteine	Sulphur	W	P	G	CE
Methionine	Sulphur	N	NP	G	E
Aspartic acid	Carboxylic	A	P	G	NE
Asparagine	Amide	N	P	G	CE
Glutamic acid	Carboxylic	A	P	G	NE
Glutamine	Amide	N	P	G	CE
Lysine	Amino	B	P	G & K	E
Arginine	Multiple amino	B	P	G	CE
Histidine	Heterocyclic	W	P	G	CE
Phenylalanine	Aromatic	N	NP	G & K	E
Tyrosine	Aromatic	W	P	G & K	CE
Tryptophan	Heterocyclic aromatic	N	NP	G & K	E
Proline	Imino	N	NP	G	CE

Abbreviations used: N, Neutral; A, Acidic; B, Basic; W, Weakly acidic or basic; P, Polar; NP, Non-polar; G, Glucogenic; K, Ketogenic; NE, Nonessential; E, Essential and CE, Conditionally essential.

Table 17.2. Estimated adult intakes of amino acids
(all values in grams per day)

ADULT	Essential amino acids required	Balance of (nonessential) amino acids required	Total protein required
Males	5.0	51.1	56.0
Females	4.5	41.5	46.0

The essential amino acids must be supplied in specific proportions.
The balance can be made up of any proportion of either essential
or nonessential amino acids. Actual intake usually exceeds these
values in most Western diets.

18
LEUCINE

Common Name

Leucine.

Alternative Names

L-Leucine.
2-Amino-4-methylvaleric acid.
Leu.
L.

Nature

Leucine is an essential, aliphatic, neutral, non-polar, ketogenic amino acid. Like isoleucine, and valine, leucine is one of the branched-chain amino acids; leucine, isoleucine and valine.

Biological Functions

- Leucine promotes protein synthesis and thus helps the healing of muscle tissue, skin and bones after traumatic injury. Branched-chain amino acids constitute one-third of the essential amino acids found in human muscle.

- Leucine may promote the formation of plasma proteins.

- Leucine increases production of growth hormones. Leucine specifically activates the synthesis of hepatocyte growth factor in the liver and helps with liver regeneration.

- Leucine helps burn visceral lipids.

- Leucine is converted to glucose more quickly than isoleucine and valine and helps to regulate blood sugar and energy levels.

- Leucine promotes glucose uptake, and α-ketoisocaproic acid, a metabolic product of leucine, also shows a similar stimulatory effect.

- However, in some people leucine may cause hypoglycemia due to its ability to stimulate insulin release from the pancreas.

- Leucine may benefit individuals with the genetic disorder phenylketonuria (PKU), who cannot metabolise the amino acid phenylalanine, by inhibiting its uptake into the brain.

- Leucine, isoleucine and valine compete with tryptophan for the same transport pathway into the brain.

- The L-isomer of leucine has no specific therapeutic role although the D-isomer is known to act as a pain killer by slowing the breakdown of the natural pain killers, the enkephalins, in the brain.

- Leucine may be decarboxylated to the alkaloid isoamylamine, a substance which has a pharmacological action on the sympathetic nervous system.

Requirement

Recommended intakes of leucine are in the range 40 to 50 mg/kg for adults. More leucine is required for growth. A leucine compendium is included for reference (Table 18.1). Good sources of leucine include corn flour, dairy products, meat, fish, beans, peas, cauliflower and nuts. Branched-chain amino acids account for around 15 to 25 percent of total protein intake in the average diet.

Toxicity

Leucine in the diet is generally nontoxic. Corn is known to contain an excess of leucine but a deficiency of tryptophan and niacin. Excess of leucine may precipitate a condition called pellagra which is associated with a deficiency of niacin, one of the B complex vitamins. This is due to the alteration in the activities of certain enzymes brought about by high levels of leucine. In the absence of niacin, the body has to use up tryptophan to try and produce enough of it. Leucine is one of the branched-chain aliphatic amino acids that may be involved in the genetic disorder resulting in maple syrup urine disease (see also isoleucine and valine).

Deficiency

In studies on young animals, a deficiency of any essential amino acid results in the growth of tiny blood vessels in the eye (corneal vascularisation). Experimental deficiency of leucine, in animals, results specifically in hypoproteinaemia (a reduction of the total plasma protein in the blood). Strict vegetarians may be at risk of leucine deficiency. Deficiency symptoms are similar to hypoglycaemia and may include dizziness and fatigue.

Table 18.1. Leucine compendium

FOOD GROUP	LEUCINE LEVEL
Milk and products	Very high
Eggs	Very high
Meat and fish	Very high
Fats and oils	Nil
Grain and products	High
Nuts and pulses	High
Root vegetables	Medium
Leaf vegetables	Medium
Fruit	Low
Sweets	Nil

19
LYSINE

Common Name

Lysine.

Alternative Names

L-Lysine.
2,6-Diaminohexanoic acid.
Lys.
K.

Nature

Lysine is an essential, basic, polar amino acid with an additional amino group on its side. It is both glucogenic and ketogenic.

Biological Functions

- Lysine may be converted into carnitine, which is an important fatty acid mobiliser and also helps lower low density lipoprotein cholesterol (LDL cholesterol).

- Lysine stimulates the release of insulin (the glucose hormone) from the pancreas.

- Lysine plays a role in the synthesis of protein in the body and promotes growth and repair of muscle.

- Lysine is essential for the formation of antibodies which protect the body against infection.

- Lysine may help to control the herpes simplex virus which causes cold sores by retarding its synthesis. It has been shown that lysine counteracts the effect of arginine which promotes the synthesis of the virus. The amino acids lysine and arginine are actively absorbed on the same transport carrier system. The rationale behind the treatment is to produce a high lysine to arginine ratio and thus reduce the rate of uptake of arginine in favour of lysine. Patients with herpes should avoid food combinations with high arginine to lysine ratios and substitute combinations with high lysine to arginine ratios. Examples of foods to be avoided include all nuts, most pulses, most grains, including rice and wheat germ, gelatin, and selected fruits and vegetables such as grapes and cabbage. Examples of food to be selected include most meat and fish, milk and yogurt, yeast, and certain fruit such as apples, apricots and figs.

- Lysine helps the body absorb calcium which is required for the development of the skeletal, nervous and hormonal systems.

- Lysine is needed to synthesise collagen which helps to maintain healthy skin, cartilage and tendons.

- Lysine promotes good appetite.

Requirement

The suggested adult intakes of lysine are around 30 to 40 mg/kg per day. A lysine compendium is included for reference (Table 19.1). Good sources of lysine include meat, fish, dairy products, beans, peas, eggs, apples and potatoes.

Toxicity

There is no common toxicity associated with lysine in the diet. Very high doses of lysine, which causes a buildup of cholesterol in the bile, may predispose toward the formation of gallstones.
High doses of lysine may lower the levels of arginine in the body because the two amino acids compete for the same transport carrier. Some people can have allergic reactions to lysine.

Deficiency

Deficiency of lysine is rare. Strict vegetarians may be at risk of lysine deficiency. A lack of lysine prevents growth in children, and may result in a loss of weight in adults. Other possible effects of deficiency include loss of appetite, tiredness and poor concentration. Lysine deficiency may be a contributing factor in hair loss in some women. Experimental deficiency, in animals, results specifically in anaemia and if prolonged may result in death.

Table 19.1. Lysine compendium

FOOD GROUP	LYSINE LEVEL
Milk and products	Very high
Eggs	High
Meat and fish	Very high
Fats and oils	Nil
Grain and products	Low
Nuts / Pulses	Low / High
Root vegetables	Medium
Leaf vegetables	Medium
Fruit	Medium
Sweets	Nil

20
PHENYLALANINE AND TYROSINE

Common Names

Phenylalanine.
Tyrosine.

Alternative Names

L-Phenylalanine.
2-Amino-3-phenylpropionic acid.
Phe.
F.

L-Tyrosine.
2-Amino-3-(4-hydroxyphenyl)-propionic acid.
Tyr.
Y.

Aromatic amino acids.

Nature

Phenylalanine is an essential, neutral, non-polar, aromatic amino acid. It is both glucogenic and ketogenic.

Tyrosine is a conditionally essential, weakly acidic, polar, aromatic amino acid. It is both glucogenic and ketogenic. Tyrosine may replace at least 70 percent of the phenylalanine requirement.

Biological Functions

- Phenylalanine is converted to tyrosine in the body. Because of this, tyrosine itself may substitute for over 70 percent of the requirement for phenylalanine. Therefore, the two amino acids are generally considered together.

- Tyrosine is converted into various neurotransmitters involved in the sympathetic nervous system. These include L-dopa, dopamine, noradrenaline and adrenaline (and also tyramine). Collectively these are called catecholamines. One route of breakdown of these products is through the enzyme called monoamine oxidase (MAO). Individuals who are on MAO-inhibitor drugs should avoid taking either phenylalanine or tyrosine rich foods.

- Tryptophan is the amino acid precursor of serotonin.

- Adrenaline itself may be further broken down to adrenochrome, a melanin-like pigment once thought to have hallucinogenic properties and to give rise to psychotic disturbances in certain susceptible individuals. This is no longer believed.

- Tyrosine may be converted to melanin, a pigment in the skin and in hair.

- Tyrosine may be converted to thyroid hormones by iodination. Iodination involves the addition of various iodide atoms to the ring structure of tyrosine. Two molecules of iodinated tyrosine must be coupled together to form thyroxine itself, one of the main thyroid hormones.

- Free phenylalanine, in the gut, may depress the appetite by releasing a hormone called cholecystokinin (CCK). Other amino acids can also have this effect, including valine, methionine and tryptophan. This results in a feeling of satiety and is the basis of the therapeutic use of phenylalanine in treating obesity.

- The D-isomer of phenylalanine has therapeutic effects in relieving pain. The L-isomer when mixed with the D-isomer results in a potent mixture called DL-phenylalanine. This also relieves pain by inhibiting the breakdown of natural pain killers, the enkephalins, in the brain (See also leucine, Chapter 18).

- Phenylalanine may improve mood in some people. Phenylalanine in normal individuals is involved in mental alertness and a feeling of well-being.

- Some individuals claim that phenylalanine has an aphrodisiac effect. Phenylalanine may give rise to phenylethylamine in the brain. It is claimed that this substance is produced by people who fall in love. (It is also found in chocolate!).

• Attention deficit hyperactivity disorder and other emotional and behavioral disorders can be triggered by too much phenylalanine in the diet.

• The branched-chain amino acids, leucine, isoleucine and valine, can inhibit the entry of phenylalanine into the brain and reduce its toxic effects on the central nervous system of people who have phenylketonurea.

Requirement

Phenylalanine is required in large amounts to form tyrosine, if the latter is not adequately supplied in the diet. The suggested intakes of phenylalanine (plus tyrosine) are around 25 to 35 mg/kg per day. A phenylalanine compendium is included for reference (Table 20.1). Good sources of phenylalanine and tyrosine are spinach, dairy products, eggs, meat, fish, potatoes, peas, nuts and bananas.

Toxicity

Doses of phenylalanine higher than 5,000 milligrams a day can cause nerve damage. If there is an excessive phenylalanine intake while the protein intake in general is low, a tyrosine toxicity may result. In experimental studies on animals, this resulted in eye problems and general signs of depression. High doses of phenylalanine should be avoided by people with diabetes and high blood pressure. Aromatic amino acid supplements should be avoided by people with melanoma, a form of skin cancer associated with excessive exposure to sunlight.

Infants and children with a genetic condition (an inborn error of metabolism) called phenylketonuria should avoid phenylalanine in the diet. This causes an intolerance to the dietary intake of phenylalanine which must be restricted to avoid mental problems. In this condition, the enzyme, phenylalanine hydroxylase, which allows phenylalanine to be converted to tyrosine is deficient and there is a buildup of unusual derivatives, some of which can cause mental retardation. After the age of 10 the brain is less sensitive to these products, but children should maintain their diets at least into their teens. The artificial sweetener, aspartame, contains 50% phenylalanine, and should be avoided by people suffering from phenylketonuria. Tyrosine can be used as a substitute for phenylalanine in the treatment of phenylketonuria.

Deficiency

Symptoms of phenylalanine deficiency include confusion, decreased alertness, faulty memory, depression, sluggish metabolism, lack of energy, reduced appetite (possibly weight loss) and vitiligo. Vitiligo develops when your skin cannot produce enough melanin pigment and patches of white skin develop. Phenylalanine deficiency results in tyrosine deficiency. Deficiency signs may include an underactive thyroid which may result in lethargy, low body temperature and weight gain.

Table 20.1. Phenylalanine plus tyrosine compendium

FOOD GROUP	PHENYLALANINE PLUS TYROSINE LEVEL
Milk and products	Very high
Eggs	Very high
Meat and fish	High
Fats and oils	Nil
Grain and products	High
Nuts and pulses	High
Root vegetables	Medium
Leaf vegetables	Medium
Fruit	Medium
Sweets	Nil

Phenylalanine and tyrosine occur in roughly equal amounts in most foods. At least 70 percent of the total aromatic amino acid requirement can be met by tyrosine.

21
VALINE

Common Name

Valine.

Alternative Names

L-Valine.
2-Amino-3-methybutyric acid.
Val.
V.

Nature

Valine is an essential, aliphatic, neutral, non-polar, ketogenic amino acid. Like leucine and isoleucine, valine, is one of the branched-chain amino acids.

Biological Functions

• Branched-chain amino acids, like valine, leucine and isoleucine, are important for their ability to generate ATP by oxidation of their carbon skeletons.

• Valine and the other branched-chain amino acids are excellent sources of energy production in skeletal muscle and serve as building blocks for muscle protein synthesis.

• Branched-chain amino acids, such as valine, serve to regulate overall nitrogen homeostasis within the brain.

• Valine is one of the amino acids that promotes the release of the gut hormone, cholecystokinin, and thereby reduces the feeling of hunger (see also phenylalanine).

- Branched-chain amino acids modulate feeding behaviors by acting on the metabolic regulatory kinase enzyme, mammalian target of rapamycin (mTOR), in the hypo-thalamus.

- Valine may be converted to isobutylamine, a substance which has a pharmacological effect on the sympathetic nervous system.

- Valine may be beneficial in cases of hepatic encephalopathy and alcohol-related brain damage.

- Branched-chain amino acids are involved in regulating the excitatory neurotransmitters, serotonin and glutamate.

- These branched-chain amino acids prevent faulty message transmission in the brain cells of people with advanced liver disease, mania, tardive dyskinesia, and possibly anorexia.

- Patients with type 2 diabetes, have impaired fasting glucose and also elevated levels of branched-chain amino acids.

- In vigorous working persons, such as athletes, depletion of muscle and plasma branched-chain amino acids is typical.

Requirement

The suggested adult intakes of valine are around 20 to 25 mg/kg per day. A valine compendium is included for reference (Table 21.1). Good sources of valine include eggs, dairy products, hazel nuts, spinach, meat, fish, cauliflower, potatoes and beans.

Toxicity

Occasionally, excessive intakes of valine cause a buildup of a metabolite called β-aminoisobutyric acid in susceptible people. This results in a general irritability, itchiness of the skin, and even psychotic disturbances (hallucinations). Such people should avoid valine-rich food and also keep histidine intakes low. Too much valine in the diet can disrupt liver and kidney function and increase the amount of ammonia in the body.

In the rare genetic disease called sickle cell anaemia, valine is substituted for glutamic acid in the haemoglobin molecule. This is not strictly a toxic effect but a genetic defect. Valine is one of the branched-chain aliphatic amino acid and may be involved in another genetic disorder called maple syrup urine disease (see also leucine and isoleucine, Chapters 18 and 22 respectively).

Deficiency

Deficiency of valine is rare. In experimental animals, a chronic deficiency of valine alone specifically results in uncoordinated movement of muscles due to issues with myelin sheaths of the neurons. Maple syrup urine disease (MSUD) is a genetic disorder in humans where the body cannot metabolise and use the essential amino acids valine, leucine and isoleucine. Sufferers produce urine that smells like maple syrup, hence the name of the disease.

Table 21.1. Valine compendium

FOOD	VALINE
Milk and products	Very high
Eggs	Very high
Meat and fish	Medium
Fats and oils	Nil
Grain and products	Medium
Nuts and pulses	Medium
Root vegetables	Medium
Leaf vegetables	Medium
Fruit	Low
Sweets	Nil

22
THREONINE

Common Name

Threonine.

Alternative Names

L-Threonine.
2-Amino-3-hydroxybutyric acid.
Thr.
T.

Nature

Threonine is an essential, hydroxylic, neutral, polar, glucogenic amino acid.

Biological Functions

- Threonine combines with aspartic acid and methionine to prevents the buildup of fat in the liver. In this regard it acts as a lipid mobilising agent.

- Threonine, in phosphoproteins, helps in the transport of phosphorous in the body.

- Threonine is important for the formation of many proteins, for example, muscle tissue, collagen, elastin and tooth enamel.

- Threonine plays an important role along with glycine and serine in porphyrin metabolism.

- Threonine supports immune system function in the production of antibodies.

- Threonine is found largely in the central nervous system, and may be helpful in treating some types of depression.

- Threonine may be useful for treatment of Lou Gehrig's Disease (Amyotrophic Lateral Sclerosis, ALS), because it increases glycine levels in the central nervous system. Glycine itself cannot cross into the central nervous system.

- Multiple Sclerosis (MS), is another disease that affects nerve and muscle function. Spasticity symptoms may be lessened with threonine supplementation.

Requirement

The suggested adult intakes of threonine are around 15 to 20 mg/kg per day. A threonine compendium is included for reference (Table 22.1). Good sources of threonine include spinach, eggs, meat, fish, cheese, cabbage, beans, apples, broccoli, brussels sprouts, peaches and tomatoes.

Toxicity

There is no common toxicity associated with threonine.

Deficiency

A general deficiency of threonine may cause irritability, confusion and personality problems. There may be a reduced resistance to infection. Other symptoms include digestion difficulties and a buildup of lipids in the liver with possible liver failure. In experimental animals, a chronic deficiency of threonine specifically results in oedema (water-logging) of various tissues.

Table 22.1. Threonine compendium

FOOD GROUP	THREONINE LEVEL
Milk and products	Very high
Eggs	Very high
Meat and fish	High
Fats and oils	Nil
Grain and products	Low
Nuts / Pulses	Low / Medium
Root vegetables	Medium
Leaf vegetables	Medium
Fruit	Low
Sweets	Nil

23
ISOLEUCINE

Common Name

Isoleucine.

Alternative Names

L-Isoleucine.
2-Amino-3-methylvaleric acid.
Ile.
I.

Nature

Isoleucine is an essential, aliphatic, neutral, polar, amino acid. It is both glucogenic and ketogenic. Like leucine, and valine, isoleucine is one of the branched-chain amino acids.

Biological Functions

- Isoleucine promotes the formation of plasma proteins, such as albumin, and also haemoglobin.

- Isoleucine is broken down for energy within muscle.

- Isoleucine also keeps energy levels stable by helping to regulate blood sugar; a deficiency of isoleucine produces symptoms similar to those of hypoglycemia.

- Isoleucine may be beneficial to brain energy metabolism because it is metabolized to the tricarboxylic acid cycle intermediate, succinyl-CoA, and the precursor, acetyl-CoA, enabling synthesis of glutamine from α-ketoglutarate and glutamate and also stimulating oxidative metabolism.

- Hyperammonaemia may inhibit tricarboxylic acid cycle activity.

Catabolism of isoleucine may help to curb this by bypassing the block as well as providing carbon skeletons for glutamate and glutamine synthesis to fixate ammonia.

- Isoleucine has a role in promoting physical and mental health.

- Branched-chain amino acids, isoleucine, leucine and valine, make up approximately one-third of muscle protein.

- Isoleucine and other branched-chain amino acid catabolism increases fatty acid oxidation and reduces the risk of obesity.

Requirement

The suggested adult intakes of isoleucine are around 15 to 20 mg/kg per day. An isoleucine compendium is included for reference (Table 23.1). Good sources of isoleucine include hazel nuts, eggs, milk, meat, fish, brussels sprouts, cauliflower, potatoes, bananas, beans, apples and peanuts.

Toxicity

Isoleucine is one of the three aliphatic amino acids with a branched chain that is broken down by the enzyme, α-keto-acid decarboxylase. See also leucine and valine. The rare deficiency of this enzyme results in a disorder called maple syrup urine disease, where there is a buildup of these acids in the blood and urine. The urine has a characteristic odour of maple syrup, hence the name of the disease which may be mild or severe depending on the degree of enzyme impairment. The amino acid is not toxic in normal individuals.

Deficiency

Deficiency of isoleucine usually only occurs in people who are deficient in dietary protein. People suffering from a number of mental and physical disorders have been found to be deficient in isoleucine. Isoleucine is essential for normal growth and for differentiation of keratinocytes and enterocytes. Deficiency of isoleucine may possibly result in an acrodermatitis enteropathica-like syndrome. Deficiency symptoms are similar to those of hypoglycaemia and may include headaches, dizziness, irritability and fatigue.

A deficiency of isoleucine, in experimental animals, specifically results in anaemia and reduced levels of the blood plasma proteins.

Table 23.1. Isoleucine compendium

FOOD GROUP	ISOLEUCINE LEVEL
Milk and products	Very high
Eggs	Very high
Meat and fish	High
Fats and oils	Nil
Grain and products	Medium
Nuts and pulses	Medium
Root vegetables	Medium
Leaf vegetables	Medium
Fruit	Low
Sweets	Nil

24
METHIONINE AND CYSTEINE

Common Names

Methionine.
Cysteine.

Alternative Names

L-Methionine.
2-Amino-4-(metylthio)butyric acid.
Met.
M.

L-Cysteine.
2-Amino-3-mercaptopropionic acid, 3-Mercaptoalanine.
Cys.
C.

Sulphur containing amino acids.

Nature

Methionine is an essential, sulphur containing (sulphydryl), neutral, non-polar, glucogenic amino acid. Cysteine may replace at least 80 percent of the methionine requirement. L-cysteine is a conditionally essential amino acid.

Biological Functions

• Methionine is converted to cysteine in the body. Cysteine itself may substitute for over 80 percent of the requirement for methionine.

• Methionine donates methyl (one-carbon, -CH_3) groups to other molecules during the synthesis of cell components. This is an important function which enables the cell to synthesise nucleic acids and other vital structures.

- Both methionine and cysteine are powerful detoxifying agents. For example, high levels of lead or copper can be removed from the body by combining with the sulphur in these amino acids.

- In another study, it was found that histamine levels in schizophrenic patients can be lowered by methionine.

- Methionine and cysteine are natural antioxidants. Methionine helps maintain the antioxidant enzyme glutathione peroxidase. Cysteine occurs in the natural antioxidant tripeptide called glutathione. In the red blood cell, together with glutathione, the glutathione peroxidase enzyme acts to destroy peroxide which is highly poisonous. This protects the membranes and various proteins from oxidation effects.

- Cysteine is converted to homocysteine in the body. Homocysteine is a pro-oxidant and requires a number of B complex vitamins, such as B_6, for its proper metabolism.

- Apart from glutathione, the sulphur-containing amino acids give rise to a number of important products in the body. These include the bile amino acid, taurine; the coenzyme, CoA; the anticoagulant, heparin; the hydrogen carrier, lipoic acid; and the B vitamin, biotin.

- Methionine protects against free radicals released by alcohol or smoking in the body. It may also protect against certain forms of radiation.

- Methionine prevents a buildup of fat in the liver. It acts as a natural lipid mobilising agent.

- Methionine may have a role in promoting the formation of plasma proteins.

- Methionine acts as a carrier of selenium (an essential trace element) in the body.

- The sulphur atoms of cysteine molecules (-SH) have the ability to link together to form a covalent bridge called the disulphide bridge (-S-S-). This occurs in many proteins to confer structural stability. Two molecules of cysteine thus joined form a compound called cystine. Conversely, cystine may be broken down to cysteine again.

- L-cysteine may up-regulate the insulin-dependent signaling cascade of glucose metabolism.

- Cysteine aids in the formation of collagen and promotes healthy skin, hair and nails.

Requirement

The suggested adult intakes of methionine plus cysteine are around 15 to 20 mg/kg per day. A methionine plus cysteine compendium is included for reference (Table 24.1). Good sources of methionine plus cysteine include brazil nuts, eggs, grapes, bread, meat, fish, bananas, spinach and rice.

Toxicity

There is no common toxicity associated with methionine. Excessive intake of any of the sulphur containing amino acids may result in elevated levels of sulphate in the urine. There may also be a tendency to flatulate. It is advisable to also take supplemental vitamin B_6 and vitamin C, when on high intakes of sulphur-containing amino acids, particularly cysteine.

Deficiency

A deficiency of methionine may cause a deficiency of choline and a buildup of fat in the liver. Experimental deficiency, in animals, results in a number of specific disturbances, including cirrhosis of the liver, kidney damage, loss of hair, anaemia, reduced levels of plasma proteins and even atherosclerosis.

One cause of cysteine deficiency is the genetic disorder homocystinuria. Cysteine is produced from methionine via a homocysteine intermediate. Defective genes for the enzyme involved, cystathionine beta synthase, can cause a buildup of homocysteine. Homocystinuria patients have to eat a carefully controlled diet low in protein to prevent homocysteine buildup and increase their intake of vitamin B_6 and B_{12} supplements and betaine. Symptoms can affect many systems, including the brain, nervous system and blood vessels. There is an increased risk of abnormal blood clotting and brittle bones.

The element sulphur itself is essential and most of the sulphur in the body occurs in the form of proteins. But, it is considered that a diet adequate in the sulphur-containing amino acids is also adequate in sulphur. Hence, a separate recommended intake for sulphur is not necessary.

Table 24.1. Methionine plus cysteine compendium

FOOD GROUP	METHIONINE PLUS CYSTEINE LEVEL
Milk and products	High
Eggs	Very high
Meat and fish	High
Fats and oils	Nil
Grain and products	High
Nuts / Pulses	Medium / Low
Root vegetables	Medium
Leaf vegetables	Medium
Fruit	Low
Sweets	Nil

Methionine and cysteine occur in equal amounts in most common foods. At least 80 percent of the sulphur amino acid requirement can be met by cysteine.

25
HISTIDINE

Common Name

Histidine.

Alternative Names

L-Histidine.
1H-imidazole-4-alanine.
α–Amino-1H-imidazole-4-propionic acid.
His.
H.

Nature

Histidine is a conditionally essential, heterocyclic, weakly basic, polar, glucogenic amino acid.

Biological Functions

- Histidine is a most active and versatile amino acid that plays multiple roles in protein interactions, and is often the key residue in enzyme catalysed reactions.

- Histidine-rich glycoprotein binds factor XIIa and inhibits contact-initiated blood clotting.

- Histidine enhances the absorption of calcium and zinc.

- Histidine-rich calcium binding protein is a regulator of sarcoplasmic reticulum Ca^{2+}-uptake, storage and release.

- Histidine may protect against some effects of radiation.

- Histidine may be involved in maintaining the integrity of the nerve covering called myelin.

- Histidine is converted into histamine in the body.

- Either substance may combine with toxic metals, such as high concentrations of copper, zinc and iron. This property has a therapeutic application in certain cases.

- Histamine itself has several physiological and pharmacological functions. It may act as a neurotransmitter in the brain.

- Histamine is involved in inflammatory processes and in tissue growth and repair. Histamine is released in response to allergic reactions and, during injury.

- Histamine produces many physical and mental side effects which can be unpleasant. Methionine may act to detoxify histamine and reduce these effects.

- Histamine also causes dilation of blood vessels in the upper body, and a reduction in blood pressure which may be of therapeutic interest.

- **Rheumatoid arthritis is correlated with relatively low levels of** histidine in the blood and increased 3-methylhistidine. Suppressor T cells have H2 receptors that can be activated by histamine. Promotion of suppressor T cell activity could be beneficial in cases of rheumatoid arthritis. Up to 6 grams of histidine per day, together with vitamin C, has been used to treat rheumatoid arthritis in some patients.

Requirement

The requirement for histidine in infants may vary from about 110 to 240 mg/day. The requirements for children are less certain, although values of 270 mg/day for younger children and 660 mg/day for older children have been suggested. Adults are capable of synthesising their own histidine and arginine requirements.

The suggested adult intakes of histidine are around 10 to 15 mg/kg per day. A histidine compendium is included for reference (Table 25.1). Good sources of histidine include meat, yogurt, cheese, lentils, eggs, peas, brussels sprouts, rice and bread.

Toxicity

Excessive intake of histidine may result in an over-production of histamine in susceptible individuals and cause flushing of the face and body. Some individuals may develop wheezing or other breathing problems. Mast cells release histamine which can trigger allergic symptoms. High levels of histamine in the brain may cause severe depression. Histidine should be avoided by women who suffer from pre-menstrual tension.

Deficiency

Adults are capable of synthesising enough histidine for normal body maintenance but, in infants, a deficiency of histidine results in poor growth and eczema. Deficiency of histidine may also cause a form of nerve deafness. Deficiency of histidine is linked with duodenal and stomach ulcers. Histamine triggers the discharge of the digestive substance that stimulates the production of gastric juices called gastrin. Without sufficient production of histamine, digestion may be impaired. Experimental deficiency of histidine, in animals, specifically results in various eye problems including the formation of cataracts and corneal vascularisation.

Table 25.1. Histidine compendium

FOOD GROUP	HISTIDINE LEVEL
Milk and products	Very high
Eggs	High
Meat and fish	Very high
Fats and oils	Nil
Grain and products	High
Nuts and pulses	Medium
Root vegetables	Medium
Leaf vegetables	Medium
Fruit	Medium, variable
Sweets	Nil

26
TRYPTOPHAN

Common Name

Tryptophan.

Alternative Names

L-Tryptophan
2-Amino-3-(3-indolyl)propionic acid.
Trp.
W.

Nature

Tryptophan is an essential, heterocyclic, aromatic, neutral, non-polar amino acid. It is both glucogenic and ketogenic.

Biological Functions

- Tryptophan may be converted to nicotinic acid (one of the B complex vitamins) in the body.

- Tryptophan may be converted to 5-hydroxytryptophan and 5-hydroxytryptamine (serotonin). Serotonin acts on smooth muscle and may cause pain sensations at nerve endings. Serotonin may also case localised oedema. Serotonin acts on the brain and may be involved in psychotic disturbs in susceptible persons.

- Serotonin may be converted to melatonin in the pineal gland in the brain. One function of melatonin is to act on melanin in the skin and cause it to concentrate, thereby causing blanching of the skin.

- Serotonin may also have an effect on the ovarian cycle.

- Serotonin levels are increased in response to carbohydrate intake. Tryptophan also causes a rise in serotonin levels, and this may serve as a therapeutic means of suppressing appetite. One of the effects of serotonin in the brain is to reduce appetite and exert a calming effect.

- Another effect of serotonin is to induce and prolong sleep. In one study it was found that 2 grams of tryptophan had a beneficial effect in this regard.

- Tryptophan may also have a therapeutic effect in treating depression. Levels of tryptophan in the brain have been associated with some forms of depression. Doses of up to 6 grams per day have been administered in severe cases.

- The concentration of tryptophan in the brain is inversely related to the levels of the neutral amino acids, leucine, isoleucine, valine, phenylalanine, tyrosine and threonine in the blood.

- Tryptophan may have an effect in reducing pain, possibly through the mechanism previously considered for D-leucine and DL-phenylalanine.

- Serotonin has a range of natural pharmacological effects in the body.

- Tryptophan may protect against some of the effects of radiation.

Requirement

The suggested adult intakes of tryptophan are around 4 to 5 mg/kg per day. A tryptophan compendium is included for reference (Table 26.1). Good sources of tryptophan include dates, eggs, sweet potatoes, spinach, kidneys, cauliflower, potatoes, milk, beans and meat.

Toxicity

Excessive intakes of tryptophan have been associated with toxicity. Tryptophan is broken down by the indole-kynurenine-niacin pathway and the serotonin-melatonin pathway giving rise to metabolites that may damage the liver. Tryptophan side effects include a higher risk of cataracts by disrupting the energy metabolism of the eye lens. Tryptophan should be avoided by persons on monoamine oxidase inhibitor (MAOI) drugs, and by women who are planning to becoming pregnant.

A tryptophan overdose can cause high levels of the type of immune cells known as eosinophils, an inflammatory connective tissue disorder called eosinophilia-myalgia syndrome, that can affect many organs and tissues and can cause severe muscle and nerve pain, fatigue and skin problems.
A tryptophan overdose can also cause serotonin syndrome, which can result in confusion, hallucinations, muscle spasms, increased sweating, fever, rapid heartbeat and diarrhea. Indeed, as with all the individual amino acids, excessive intakes of supplements of them are inadvisable as prolonged high intakes of several of them are now associated with toxicity. In animal studies, high levels of tryptophan caused inflammation in lungs, leg muscles and other organs.

Deficiency

Experimental deficiency of tryptophan, in animals, specifically results in a number of disturbances including cataracts, poor teeth, loss of hair, reproductive problems, and gastric disturbances. Pellagra can be caused by decreased intake of niacin or tryptophan. Tryptophan deficiency can result in dermatitis, and digestive problems. Emotional effects of tryptophan deficiency may include difficulty sleeping, withdrawal from social life, low self-esteem, depression and even dementia.

Table 26.1. Tryptophan compendium

FOOD GROUP	TRYPTOPHAN LEVEL
Milk and products	High
Eggs	Very high
Meat and fish	Medium
Fats and oils	Nil
Grain and products	Medium
Nuts and pulses	Medium
Root vegetables	Medium
Leaf vegetables	Low
Fruit	Low
Sweets	Nil

27
ARGININE

Common Name

Arginine.

Alternative Names

L-Arginine.
2-Amino-5-guanidinovaleric acid.
Arg.
R.

Nature

Arginine is a conditionally essential, basic, polar, glucogenic amino acid with a multiple amino (guanidino) group on its side chain. L-Arginine contains 32% nitrogen.

Biological Functions

• Arginine is converted to ornithine in the body, and hence urea. As such, arginine acts as an important detoxifying agent.

• Arginine promotes the transport of amino acids into the cells and stimulates protein regeneration.

• Nitric oxide (NO), an important signaling molecule in the body, is produced from arginine. Up to 40% of ingested arginine is broken down by the intestines and liver, reducing the amount available for nitric oxide production. However, another amino acid, citrulline, circumvents this breakdown, and is converted to arginine in the kidneys, and thus increases nitric oxide production.

• Seminal fluid is made up of about 80 percent arginine. Some susceptible males may require supplementary arginine for adequate production of sperm. Doses of up to 8 grams of arginine per day have been used to treat infertility.

- The relationship between arginine and lysine in the control of herpes simplex was previously considered in the chapter on lysine.

- Arginine is important in the immune system. It has been found to stimulate the thymus gland and promote healing in some animal experiments.

- Manganese increases the uptake of arginine.

- Elevation of certain amino acids in the blood stimulates the release of the pituitary hormone, somatotropin. Arginine and ornithine are particularly potent in this regard and work best during sleep. This may have a therapeutic application in body building and weight reduction.

- The release of another hormone, insulin, from the pancreas, is also stimulated by several amino acids. The amino acids may be listed as follows in decreasing order of potency: arginine, lysine, phenylalanine, leucine, methionine, valine, histidine, threonine and tryptophan, respectively. It has been found that arginine, in combination with either phenylalanine or leucine, is particularly potent in this regard.

Requirement

The requirements for arginine are unknown. An estimated arginine requirement for infants based on the composition of human milk and the known requirements for other essential amino acids is probably in the range 25 to 50 mg/kg body weight, with an average value near 40 mg/kg, or about 280 mg/day. Arginine, like histidine, does not appear to be essential for normal adults. An arginine compendium is included for reference (Table 27.1). Good sources of arginine include nuts, beans, peas, cabbage, rice, cucumber, grapes, oranges, meat and fish.

Toxicity

Excessive arginine (and glutamine, another amino acid), may be associated with catatonic states in susceptible individuals. The mechanism is unknown, however. Schizophrenics should therefore avoid arginine supplements.

Deficiency

Adults are capable of synthesising enough arginine for normal body maintenance, but infants require arginine in their diet for normal growth. Experimental deficiency of arginine, in male animals, specifically results in a reduced production of sperm. Deficiency of arginine also reduces glucose tolerance (insulin production), and lipid metabolism in the liver of experimental animals. Cholesterol levels may be elevated.

Table 27.1. Arginine compendium

FOOD GROUP	ARGININE LEVEL
Milk and products	Low
Eggs	Medium
Meat and fish	Medium
Fats and oils	Nil
Grain and products	Medium
Nuts and pulses	Very high
Root vegetables	Medium
Leaf vegetables	High, variable
Fruit	Low
Sweets	Nil

28
PROTEIN QUALITY

Before leaving the proteins, some consideration of protein quality is appropriate. Typical overall protein intakes have been specified. These values do not specify the protein quality but corrections include values for suboptimal quality, incomplete digestion and some individual variation. Appropriate intakes for each of the essential amino acids have also been specified. It is also assumed that there is an overall adequate energy intake which included some carbohydrate to spare glucose formation from the glucogenic amino acids. As a general rule, total energy intake should be at least one and a half times the basal metabolic rate to maintain nitrogen balance (or around 400 kJ per gram of protein in the minimum diet).

For any given protein, a value called quality can be calculated from a consideration of its essential amino acid composition. The better the balance of all the essential amino acids in a protein, the better is its quality. If a protein is deficient, even in only one of these amino acids, then its overall quality is lowered. The reason for this derives from the fact that the body needs the correct variety of different amino acids in order to sythesise proteins. If a particular amino acid is missing the cell cannot go ahead and synthesise the other parts of the protein and then, when the missing amino acid is supplied at a later date, join up the various pieces to form the complete protein. In fact, in these limiting circumstances, none of the other amino acids that are supplied in the diet are available for protein synthesis. Instead, they are generally converted to carbohydrate and lipid (to provide energy), with the removal of their nitrogen which is excreted resulting in a negative nitrogen balance. The only way to reverse this negative balance is to supply the missing amino acid itself or another protein which does contain it, at the same time as the poor-quality protein. Some proteins are more complete than others.

In the early days, it was generally considered that proteins from animal sources were complete, whereas proteins from plant sources were incomplete. It was said that animals provided first class proteins and plants provided second class proteins. This oversimplification is no longer held. There are many exceptions. Furthermore, by mixing two incomplete proteins, it is possible to end up with an effectively complete combined protein diet, even if the diet is limited to vegetable sources only. Different levels of each amino acid occur in each protein source. So, the overall diet determines the overall intake at any given meal. Second, even if only a single source of protein is consumed, it does not follow that the full complement of its amino acids will be available for protein synthesis in the body. Nowadays, there are very precise definitions of protein quality. Suffice it, here, to define three of the more commonly used estimates of protein quality.

Amino Acid Ratios

The ratio methods express the nitrogen content of the essential amino acids in a protein to the total nitrogen content of the protein. This method takes no account of the distribution of amino acids or their digestibility. The ratio may be expressed either as a percentage (relative value) or as an absolute value. In top quality proteins, the absolute ratio should be around 3 or higher, in low quality proteins the ratio is around 2 or less. Milk protein (bovine), has a value of 3.25. Eggs have a value of 3.22. On the other hand, gelatin has a value of only 1.31.

Net Protein Utilisation (Biological Value Scales)

These scales express the nitrogen which is retained as a percent of either the total nitrogen absorbed from the diet (biological value), or the total nitrogen provided in the diet (net protein utilisation). The biological value scale takes no account of the unavailable nitrogen during digestion. The net protein utilisation scale does account for this factor and is, therefore, a better nutritive measure. Protein quality depends on both the structural completeness and the availability (digestibility and absorbability) if its amino acids.

Amino Acid Scores (Chemical Scores)

The amino acid score (or chemical score) method compares the content of each essential amino acid with the content of a reference protein. A reference protein is a protein with a known (or specified) essential amino acid composition which meets the requirement for a particular species or physiological state. Reference proteins are non-limiting. In the past, the reference proteins most frequently used were hen's egg protein or cow's milk protein, which are both excellent examples of complete protein, and are used with 90 - 100% efficiency on low intakes. Some authors still use these references. However, the concept of a theoretically perfect protein, which is used with 100% efficiency at whatever level it is fed in the diet, has been developed over the years. Such perfect proteins may also be used (or designed) as a means of expressing recommended daily intakes.

For example, in 1973, a hypothetical reference protein was defined which is frequently used to calculate score patterns. Provided the amino acid composition of a given protein is known this is a very simple method to use and gives a value known as the chemical score. This is defined as the limiting essential amino acid content expressed as a percentage of the corresponding reference value. For example, the reference value for methionine is 3.5. If methionine is the limiting amino acid in a certain protein, say with a value of 2.8. Then the chemical score is given as 80. The results for most amino acids are straightforward. However, the values given for methionine and phenylalanine underestimate the quality as they do not take into account the possible contribution of cysteine and tyrosine, respectively.

Reference proteins may also be used as alternative theoretical high quality proteins. For example, the 1974 reference protein is designed to provide all the essential amino acids in optimum proportions. Top quality proteins should have no limiting amino acid and consequently a nominal amino acid score of 100. The essential amino acid patterns in various reference proteins are given in Table 28.1.

Various authors use different methods. The values obtained using the three methods are similar but not identical as shown in Table 28.2. But the differences are in most cases only of academic interest. In general, high quality proteins (on all scales) include the animal proteins of milk, eggs, meat and fish, and certain grains and pulses such as rice and soya beans. Gelatin is an exception being a very poor quality protein of animal origin. Lower quality proteins include mainly vegetable proteins such as some grains and pulses, nuts and fruit. It should be noted that some vegetables and fruit contain insignificant amounts of protein. As explained above, only the limiting amino acid determines the extent to which all the other amino acids can be used. Thus, a given source, (for example, corn), may be low in lysine but rich in leucine. In this case, much of the leucine is wasted unless other proteins with complementary amounts of lysine are consumed at the same time. For protein synthesis to occur, all the required amino acids must be present at the site of protein synthesis in adequate amounts at the same time. This alone is sufficient reason to advocate a mixed and varied diet at all times. Many vegetables are low in lysine, methionine, tryptophan or threonine. Pulses are low in methionine but rich in lysine and threonine. Wheat, rice, oats, millet and sesame seeds are limited by lysine and possible also by methionine and threonine. Fruit is generally low in all amino acids except lysine. Gelatin itself is low in several essential amino acids including valine, tyrosine and cysteine, and it does not contain tryptophan. An important feature of vegetable proteins is their ability to complement each other. For example, by combining pulses which are low in methionine with grains which are low in lysine it is possible to provide a high quality meal which is adequate in all the essential amino acids. It is the job of the dietician to plan such combinations in the light of economic necessity, local availability of produce, individual taste and possible health disorders. Some traditional examples of excellent complementation include Italian macaroni and cheese, Irish vegetable stew, and Chinese chicken chow-mein.

There is another way of looking at quality. Assume that a person had to survive on a single source of protein. Then, how much of this protein would be required. It can be shown that different daily amounts of different types of protein are required. The less the amount required the higher the quality of a particular protein. For such a comparison, it is convenient to specify the amount which will just prevent a negative nitrogen balance from occurring as the minimum daily amount required. In these circumstances, about 20 grams of egg protein has the same effect as 25 grams of milk protein, or 30 grams of potato protein, or 40 grams of white flour protein, or 65 grams of whole wheat bread protein. But no amount of pure gelatin will prevent a negative nitrogen balance, even if provided with adequate carbohydrate, lipid and other nutrients. This is because several essential amino acids are deficient and tryptophan is missing altogether. Unless the protein is of extremely low quality (as with prolonged diets on very limited vegetable sources), the general suggested minimum values are perfectly sufficient. In fact, these values refer to the values for an average protein diet of quality around 70 percent. The absolute minimum daily value for adults on the highest quality protein is around 0.5 g/kg. Sometimes even lower values have been quoted. The actual intake of protein, on the other hand, in the typical Western diet is greater than any of the suggested values and frequently exceeds three times the appropriate minimum. Much remains to be done in this important field. Table 28.3 gives the average distribution of essential amino acids in a typical Western mixed protein diet. Interestingly, about half the amino acid content consists of various essential amino acids. The other half consists of the nonessential amino acids. The amino acid chemical score for such a mixture, relative to the 1973 reference protein, comes out at 100 percent.

Table 28.1. Essential amino acid patterns in various reference proteins (all values in grams per 100 protein)

Essential Amino Acid	Maintenance pattern (1949)	Reference pattern (1957)	Score pattern (1973)	Alternative high quality pattern (1974)	Gelatin
Leucine	4.3	4.9	7.0	7.0	2.9
Lysine	3.2	4.3	5.4	5.1	4.0
Phenylalanine	4.3	2.9	6.1	7.3	2.1
Tyrosine	---	2.9	---	a	0.3
Valine	3.2	4.3	5.0	4.8	2.2
Threonine	1.9	2.8	4.0	3.5	1.9
Isoleucine	2.8	4.3	4.0	4.2	1.4
Methionine	4.3	2.3	3.5	2.6	0.8
Cysteine	---	2.0	---	b	Trace
Histidine	0.0	---	---	1.7	0.6
Tryptophan	1.0	1.4	1.0	1.1	0.0
Arginine	0.0	---	---	---	7.8

a. Tyrosine is included in the phenylalanine value.

b. Cysteine is included in the methionine value.

It can be assumed that every 100 g protein contains 16 g nitrogen. The 1957 protein is a relatively low quality protein, whereas the 1974 alternative reference protein is a high quality protein (similar to the 1973 pattern). Gelatin, a very low quality protein, is included for comparison only. Generally, most proteins in each food group such as meat, fish, dairy products and grains, have their own characteristic amino acid patterns. For example, most grains are low in lysine.

Table 28.2. Comparison of three methods of estimating protein quality

PROTEIN SOURCE	METHOD		
	Relative value	Net protein utilisation	Chemical score
Human milk	96	94	100
Hen's eggs	99	87	100
Cow's milk	98	81	95
Soya beans	79	67	74
Rice	80	63	67
Millet	85	44	63
Wheat	86	49	53
Corn	62	36	49

In general, it may be assumed that 100 grams of protein contain 16 grams of nitrogen. Alternatively, every 1 g nitrogen corresponds to 6.25 g protein. But there are slight variations. The factor 6.25 holds well for eggs, meat and fish, and many pulses, fruits and vegetables. The factor 6.38 is better for milk. Some nuts, and vegetables have factors ranging from 6.25 to 5.30. For example, most nuts and seeds have values from 5.46 to 5.30 (almonds are exceptional at 5.18), and most grains have values around 5.95 to 5.83 (bran itself is exceptional at 6.31). Pure gelatin has the value 5.55.

Table 28.3. Average distribution of amino acids in a typical mixed protein diet (in grams per 100 grams protein).

Amino Acid	Content
Leucine	7.7
Lysine	6.4
Phenylalanine	4.8
Tyrosine	3.5
Valine	5.6
Threonine	4.2
Isoleucine	4.4
Methionine	2.3
Cysteine	1.8
Histidine	2.8
Tryptophan	1.4
Arginine	5.1

Total aromatic amino acids 8.3, and total Sulphur-containing amino acids 4.1. The total of the above essential amino acids comes to fifty percent. The remaining fifty percent consists of all the other (non-essential) amino acids, of which glutamic acid alone accounts for some 20 percent.

A1

Solid and Liquid Portions Commonly Used in Cooking and Dietetics

The commercial unit of volume for fluids is the gallon. In the US the gallon has a volume of 3,785 ml approximately, whereas in the U.K. the gallon has a volume of 4,546 ml approximately. In the US the commercial unit of volume for dry substances is the bushel which has a volume of 35,239 ml approximately. Therefore, the bushel is just over 9.3 times the volume of the US gallon. In the U.K. the bushel is simply 8 gallons (or 36,369 ml approximately), and the gallon also serves as the commercial unit of volume for dry substances.

Further confusion arises when dry substances are expressed as dry pints, which are defined as one-eighth of a gallon and therefore have a volume of 551 ml approximately, as compared to 473 ml approximately, for the liquid pint, in the US Again, liquids because of their different densities have different weights per unit volume. For example, 100 ml liquid may weigh anything from about 90 to 150 grams.

Domestic measures expressed in terms of cups or spoons are also notoriously ambiguous. Most of these measures are related to simple multiples or fractions of the fluid ounce or the dry ounce. Unfortunately, the definition of the ounce itself varies (because the ounce is defined as 1/160th of a gallon, which has two definitions). Also the multiples and fractions used by different authors may also vary. For example, the teacup has a defined capacity of 8 fluid ounces whereas the breakfast cup contains 10 fluid ounces. Both of these measures are in current use. The term small teaspoon is occasionally used in the U.K. The small teaspoon contains one-eighth of a fluid ounce whereas the (level) standard teaspoon contains one-sixth of a fluid ounce. Expressed in ml, therefore, the capacity of a teaspoon may be either 3.55 or 4.74 ml. But such accuracy is meaningless and in the Table A1.1 the rounded value of 4 ml has been used for the U.K. measure. Similar considerations have been applied to some of the other measures listed.

Thankfully, this confusing state of affairs is coming to an end. With the advent of International System of Units, recent texts are getting around to express all measures in units of mass and volume which are derived from the basic SI units, that is the kilogram and the litre (or more strictly the cubic decimetre), respectively.

SI Units

The *Système International d'Unités* (SI) or International System of Units is the official name for the metric system. SI units are used in this book

The three units of this system most often used in nutrition are the unit of mass called the kilogram, kg, the unit of volume called the litre, l, and the unit of energy called the joule, J. These units are related to the older units such as the International pound, lb, the Imperial pint, pt, and the thermochemical calorie, cal, approximately, as follows:

$$1 \text{ kg} = 2.205 \text{ lb}$$
$$1 \text{ l} = 1.760 \text{ pt}$$
$$1 \text{ J} = 0.239 \text{ cal}$$

Conversely, the old units are related to the SI units as follows:

$$1 \text{ lb} = 0.454 \text{ kg}$$
$$1 \text{ pt} = 0.568 \text{ l}$$
$$1 \text{ cal} = 4.184 \text{ J (exactly)}$$

Further details are given in Table A1.1. The SI system also has special names for very large or very small amounts. The multiple kilo, k, represents one thousand: for example, kg represents 1000 grams and kJ represents 1000 joules. The multiple mega, M, represents one million: for example, MJ represents one million joules (or 1,000 kJ). The submultiple milli, m, represents one thousandth, for example, mg represents 0.001 grams and ml represents 0.001 litres. For vitamins and trace elements the submultiple micro, μ (less preferably mc), must be used. This represents one millionth, for example, mg represents 0.000001 grams. It is easy to remember that there are:

$$1000\ \mu g\ =\ 1\ mg$$
$$1000\ mg\ =\ 1\ g$$
$$1000\ g\ =\ 1\ kg$$

Table A1.1. Solid and liquid portions commonly used in cooking and dietetics

PORTION	EQUIVALENT VALUE (some approximate)			
SOLIDS	(grams)			
Stone	6,350	(Avoirdupois)		
Kilogram	1,000			
Pound	454	(Avoirdupois, or International)		
Dry cup	200 – 50	variable		
Average serving	113			
Standard portion	100			
Ounce	28	(Avoirdupois)		
Tablespoon	15 – 4	variable		
Dessertspoon	10 – 3	variable		
Dry teaspoon	5 – 2	variable		
Gram	1			
LIQUIDS	(millilitres)			
Gallon	4,546	(Imperial)	3,785	(in US)
Quart	1,136	(Imperial)	946	(in US)
Litre	1,000			
Pint	568	(Imperial)	473	(in US)
Measuring cup	284	(in UK)	237	(in US)
Gill	142	(Imperial)	118	(in US)
Standard volume	100			
Fluid ounce	28	(Imperial)	30	(in US)
Tablespoon	14	(in UK, variable)	15	(in US, variable)
Dessertspoon	7	(in UK, variable)	10	(in US, variable)
Teaspoon	4	(in UK, variable)	5	(in US, variable)
Millilitre	1			

A2

Some Individual Fatty Acids

Structural Code

Fatty acid formulae may be expressed according to the number of carbon atoms followed by the number of double bonds. For example, oleic acid which contains 18 carbon atoms and one double bond may be written in shorthand as C18:1. Unless otherwise indicated, all double bonds are in the *cis* form, and all fatty acids are straight-chained. A *trans* double bond is indicated by the letter t. A branched chain is indicated by the letters br. Hydroxy acids and keto acids may be indicated by the letters OH and k, respectively. The position of each double bond may also be indicated in parenthesis, where the positions are numbered from the carboxyl end of the molecule. Thus, oleic acid may be written in full as C18:1 (9). In some cases, where there are mixed *cis* and *trans* double bonds in the same molecule, each double bond may be qualified by adding the letter c or t to the number in parenthesis.

Table A2.1.i. Some of the main naturally occurring fatty acids

COMMON NAME	STRUCTURAL CODE	CHEMICAL NAME
Saturated acids		
Formic	C1:0	Methanoic
Acetic	C2:0	Ethanoic
Propionic	C3:0	Propanoic
Lactic	OH-C3:0	Hydroxypropanoic
Pyruvic	k-C3:0	Ketopropanoic
Butyric	C4:0	Butanoic
Isobutyric	br-C4:0	Methylpropanoic
Valeric	C5:0	Pentanoic
alpha-Methylbutyric	br-C5:0	2- Methylbutanoic
Isovaleric	br-C5:0	3-Methylbutanoic
Caproic	C6:0	Hexanoic
Caprylic	C8:0	Octanoic
Capric	C10:0	Decanoic
Lauric	C12:0	Dodecanoic
Myristic	C14:0	Tetradecanoic
Hydroxymyristic	OH-C14:0	3-Hydroxytetradecanoic
Pentadecyclic	C15:0	Pentadecanoic
Palmitic	C16:0	Hexadecanoic
Margaric	C17:0	Heptadecanoic
Stearic	C18:0	Octadecanoic
alpha-Hydroxystearic	OH-C18:0	2-Hydroxyoctadecanoic
Tuberculostearic	br-C19:0	10-Methyloctadecanoic
Arachidic	C20:0	Eicosanoic
Phytanic	br-C20:0	3,7,11,15-Tetramethylhexadecanoic
Behenic	C22:0	Docosanoic
-----	OH-C23:0	2-Hydroxytricosanoic
Lignoceric	C24:0	Tetracosanoic
Cerebronic	OH-C24:0	2-Hydroxytetracosanoic
Cerotic	C26:0	Hexacosanoic
Montanic	C28:0	Octacosanoic
Melissic	C30:0	Triacontanoic
Micoceranic	br-C31:0	2,4, 6-Trimethyloctacosanoic
Lacceroic	C32:0	Dotriacontanoic
Gheddic	C34:0	Tetratriacontanoic
Ceroplastic	C36:0	Pentatriacontanoic

Continued /

Table A2.1.ii.

COMMON NAME	STRUCTURAL CODE	CHEMICAL NAME

Monounsaturated acids

COMMON NAME	STRUCTURAL CODE	CHEMICAL NAME
Acrylic	C3:1	Propenoic
Crotonic	t-C4:1 (2)	*trans*-2-Butenoic
Tiglic	br-C5:1 (2)	*cis*-2-Methyl-2-butenoic
Isohydroascorbic	C6:1 (2)	*cis*-2-Hexenoic
Obtusilic	C10:1 (4)	*cis*-4-Decenoic
Caproleic	C10:1 (9)	*cis*-9-Decenoic
Linderic	C12:1 (4)	*cis*-4-Dodecenoic
Lauroleic	C12:1 (9)	*cis*-9-Dodecenoic
Tsuzic	C14:1 (4)	*cis*-4-Tetradecenoic
Physeteric	C14:1 (5)	*cis*-5-Tetradecenoic
Myristoleic	C14:1 (9)	*cis*-9-Tetradecenoic
-----	t-C16:1 (3)	*trans*-3-Hexadecenoic
Palmitoleic	C16:1 (9)	*cis*-9-Hexadecenoic
Palmitvaccenic	C16:1 (11)	*cis*-11-Hexadecenoic
Petroselinic	C18:1 (6)	*cis*-6-Octadecenoic
Oleic	C18:1 (9)	*cis*-9-Octadeoenoic
Elaidic	t-C18:1 (9)	*trans*-9-Octadecenoic
Ricinoleic	OH-C18:1 (9)	12-Hydroxy-*cis* -9-Octadecenoic
cis-Vaccenic	C18:1 (11)	*cis*-11-Octadecenoic
trans-Vaccenic	t-C18:1 (11)	*trans*-11-Octadecanoic
-----	C18:1 (12)	*cis*-12-Octadecenoic
Gadoleic	C20:1 (9)	*cis*-9-Eicosenoic
Gondoic	C20:1 (11)	*cis*-11-Eicosenoic
Cetoleic	C22:1 (11)	*cis*-11-Docosenoic
Erucic	C22:1 (13)	*cis*-l3-Docosenoic
Brassidic	t-C22:1 (13)	*trans*-13-Docosenoic
Nervonic (Selacholeic)	C24: 1 (15)	*cis*-15-Tetracosenoic
Hydroxynervonic	OH-C24:1 (15)	2-Hydroxy-*cis*-15-Tetracosenoic
Ximenic	C26:1 (17)	*cis*-17-Hexacosenoic
Lumequeic	C30:1 (21)	*cis*-21-Triacontenoic

Continued /

Table A2.1.iii.

COMMON NAME	STRUCTURAL CODE	CHEMICAL NAME

Polyunsaturated acids

Dienoic

Sorbic	C6:2(2,4)	all-*cis*-2,4-Hexadienoic
-----	C16:2 (7,10)	all-*cis*-7,10-Hexadecadienoic
-----	C16:2(9,12)	all-*cis*-9,12-Hexadecadienoic
-----	C18:2 (6,9)	all-*cis*-6,9-Octadecadienoic
Linoleic (LA)	C18:2 (9,12)	all-*cis*-9,12-Octadecadienoic
Linoelaidic	tt-C18:2 (9,12)	all-*trans*-9,12-Octadecadienoic
-----	tt-C18:2 (10,12)	all-*trans*-10,12-Octadecadienoic
-----	C20:2 (11,14)	all-*cis*-11,14-Eicosadienoic
-----	C22:2 (13,16)	all-*cis*-13,16-Docosadienoic

Trienoic

Hiragonic	C16:3(6,10,14)	all-*cis*-6,10,14-Hexadecatrienoic
-----	C16:3(7,10,13)	all-*cis*-7,10,13-Hexadecatrienoic
γ-Linolenic (GLA)	C18:3 (6,9,12)	all-*cis*-6,9,12-Octadecatrienoic
Punicic	C18:3 (9c,11t,13c)	*cis*-9-*trans*-11-*cis*-3-Octadecatrienoic
α-Eleostearic	C18:3 (9c,11t,13t)	*cis*-9-*trans*-11-*trans*-13-Octadecatrienoic
β-Eleostearic	ttt-C18:3(9,11,13)	all-*trans*-9,11,13-Octodecatrienoic
α-Linolenic (ALA)	C18:3 (9,12,15)	all-*cis*-9,12,15-Octadecatrienoic
Linolenelaidic	ttt-C18: 3 (9,12,15)	all-*trans*-9,12,15-Octadecatrienoic
Dihomo-γ-Linolenic (Mead acid) (DGLA)	C20:3 (8,11,14)	all-*cis*-8,11,14-Eicosatrienoic

Continued /

Table A2.1.iv.

COMMON NAME	STRUCTURAL CODE	CHEMICAL NAME
Tetraenoic		
-----	C16:4(4,7,10,13)	all-*cis*-4,7,10,13- Hexadecatetraenoic
Stearidonic (SDA)	C18:4 (4,8,12,15)	all-*cis*-4,8,12,15- Octadecatetraenoic
alpha-Parinaric	C18:4(9,11,13,15)	all-*cis*-9,11,13,15- Octadecatetraenoic
Arachidonic (AA)	C20:4 (5,8,11,14)	all-*cis*-5,8,11,14- Eicosatetraenoic
Pentaenoic		
Timnodonic	C20:5 (5,8,11,14,17)	all-*cis*-5,8,11,14,17- Eicosapentaenoic (EPA)
Clupanodonic	C22:5 (4,8,12,15,19)	all-*cis*-4,8,12,15,19- Docosapentaenoic (DPA)
Hexaenoic		
Docosahexaenoic	C22:6 (4,7,10,13,16,19)	all-*cis*-4,7,10,13,16,19- Docosahexaenoic (DHA)
Nisinic	C24:6 (4,8,12,15,18,21)	all-*cis*-4,8,12,15,18,21- Tetracosahexaenoic

Omega Convention

Sometimes, fatty acids are classified according to the omega convention. This convention is explained in the following text.

The omega convention classifies unsaturated fatty acids according to the location of the double bonds as measured from the non-carboxyl end of the molecule. For example, linoleic acid has 18 carbon atoms and two double bonds located at carbon numbers 9 and 12 respectively as counted from the carboxyl end. Hence, the structural code may be written as C18:2 (9,12). But counting from the opposite or omega end, these double bonds will be said to be located at positions n-6 and n-9, respectively. This is because in this example the total number of carbon atoms (n) equals 18; so 18 - 6 equals 12, and 18 - 9 equals 9. Therefore, in the omega code, the molecule can be written as C18:2 (n-6,9). Synthetic fatty acids generally do not have common names.

None of the acids in Table A2.2 occur in nature. But all those with essential fatty acid activity give rise to prostaglandins in the body, hence may be considered as drugs. An interesting structural feature which is common to many of the active fatty acids is the occurrence of double bonds in the omega 6 and 9 positions. Interestingly, linoleic, linolenic, dihomo-γ-linolenic and arachidonic acids all have this same feature in common and all have 100 percent activity on the scale used in Table A2.2. It is now believed the any fatty acid capable of being converted to a C19:4, C20:4, or C21:4 acid with the key double bond structure (5,8,11,14) from the carboxyl end, will have essential fatty acid activity and be capable of forming an active prostaglandin in the body.

Table A2.2. Relative essential fatty acid activity or biopotency
of synthetic fatty acids

FATTY ACID STRUCTURE

STRUCTURAL CODE [1]	OMEGA CLASSIFICATION	NOMINAL VALUE (percent activity)
C20:4 (5,8,11,14)	(n-6,9,12,15)	140
C22:5 (4,7,10,13,16)	(n-6,9,12,15,18)	140
C18:3 (6,9,12)	(n-6,9,12)	115
C17:2 (9,12)	(n-5,8)	100
C18:2 (9,12)	(n-6,9)	100
C20:3 (8,11,14)	(n- 6,9,12)	100|
C21:4 (5,8,11,14)	(n-7,10,13,16)	70, variable
C21:3 (8,11,14)	(n-7,10,13)	55
C19:4 (5,8,11,14)	(n-5,8,11,14)	50
C20:2 (11,14)	(n-6,9)	45
C18:4 (6,9,12,15)	(n-3,6,9,12)	39
C19:3 (8,11,14)	(n-5,8,11)	25, variable
C19:3 (10,13)	(n-6,9)	10
C18:1 (12)	(n-6)	0, variable
C18:3 (8,11,14)	(n-4,7,10)	0
C18:4 (5,8,11,14)	(n-4,7,10,13)	0
C19:3 (7,10,13)	(n-6,9,12)	0
C20:3 (7,10,13)	(n-7,10,13)	0
C22:3 (8,11,14)	(n-8,11,14)	0

1. For details of the structural code used above see Table A2.1.

A3

Common Toxicity and Deficiency Symptoms of Macronutrients

Table A3.1i. Toxicity and deficiency symptoms of macronutrients

MACRONUTRIENT	TOXICITY	DEFICIENCY
Water	Oedema. High blood pressure. Nausea Dilution of electrolytes, e.g. sodium (hyponatremia). Cell swelling. Muscle weakness. Increased intracranial pressure. Confusion. Slow heartbeat.	Dehydration. Thirst. Renal failure. Confusion. Increased cholesterol. Elevated blood pressure. Buildup of toxins. Skin disorders.
(Oxygen)	Lung irritation. Convulsions.	Irreversible cell damage. Death.
(Energy)	Obesity and related disorders.	Weight loss.
Carbohydrate	Obesity. May potentiate diabetes. Coma.	Weight loss. Ketosis. Coma.
Dietary Fibre	Nausea. Diarrhoea. Flatulence. Decreased mineral absorption, e.g., calcium, magnesium, iron and zinc. Dehydration. Lower cholesterol.	Bowel disorders. Constipation. Diverticulosis. Colon cancer risk. Gallstones. Blood glucose fluctuations.

Continued /

Table A3.1ii.

MACRONUTRIENT	TOXICITY	DEFICIENCY
Lipid	Obesity. Indigestion. Possibly bowel disease. Risk of colon cancer. Toxicity of fat-soluble vitamins, e.g., A and D.	Weight loss. Poor growth. Skin lesions. Negative nitrogen balance. Lack of fat-soluble vitamins, e.g., A and D. Vision problems.
Essential Fatty Acids	Non-toxic from food.	Dermatitis. Change in body fatty acid composition. Increased cholesterol. Possible weight loss. Impaired brain function.
Protein	Obesity. Acidosis. High blood pressure. Risk of kidney failure.	Weight loss. Net nitrogen loss. Poor growth. Slow healing. Irregular menstruation. Enlarged fatty liver. Low immune response. Fluid imbalance. Kwashiorkor. Marasmus.
Essential Amino Acids	Non-toxic from food.	Poor growth. Slow healing. Net nitrogen loss. Risk of infection. Malabsorption. Muscle wasting. Dull skin. Lackluster hair. Nervousness. Lethargy. Fatigue.

Bibliography

General reading

Bryce-Smyth, D. and Hodgkinson, L. (1986). The zinc solution, Century Arrow.

Burkitt, D. (1982). Don't forget the fibre in your diet, Third edition, Martin Dunitz.

Candlish, J. (1981). Metabolic water and the camel's hump—a textbook survey, *Biochemical Education* 9(3) 1981 96-97.

Cathie, K. (1976). The complete calorie counter, Pan Books.

Cathie, K. (1978). The complete carbohydrate counter, Pan Books.

Chaitow, L. (1985). Amino acids in therapy, Thorsons.

Forbes, A. (1990). Healthy eating: cooking with vitamins and minerals, Penguin Books.

Graham, J. and Odent, M. (1986). The Z factor, Thorsons.

Lewis, A. (1983). Selenium, Revised Expanded Edition Thorsons.

Mervyn, L. (1981). The B vitamins, Thorsons.

Mervyn, L. (1981). Vitamin C, Thorsons.

Mervyn, L. (1984). Vitamin E, Revised Edition, Nature's Way Series, Thorsons.

Mervyn, L. (1984). Vitamins A, D, K, Nature's Series, Thorsons.

Sherman, A. (1984). The sodium counter, Arlington Books.

Thomas, J. (1985). The fat counter, Pan Books.

Trimmer, E. (1987). The magic of magnesium, Thorsons.

Tudge, C. (1985). The food connection, BBC Publication.

Wright, M. (1984). The salt counter, Pan Books.

Encyclopedias and Dictionaries

Adrian, J., Legrand, G and Frange, R. (1988). Dictionary of food and nutrition. Translator, B. Weitz. Translation Editors, E. Rolfe, I. Morton and L. Mabbit Ellis Horwood.

Black's agricultural dictionary, (1981). Edited by D. B. Dalal-Clayton Adam and Charles Black, Black Publishers Ltd.

Butterworth' s dictionary of nutrition and food technology, (1982). Edited by A. E. Bender, Butterworths.

Campion, K. (1986). Vegetarian encyclopedia, Century paperbacks.

Fischer, R. B. (1986). A dictionary of diets, slimming and nutrition, Paladin.

Illustrated Stedman's medical dictionary, (1982). 24th Edition, Williams and Wilkins.

Kirschmann, J. D. (1979). Nutrition almanac, Revised Fourth Edition, McGraw-Hill.

Mayes, A. (1986). The dictionary of nutritional health: guide to the relation between diet and health, Thorsons.

McGraw-Hill Encyclopedia of food, agriculture and nutrition, (1977). Edited by D. N. Lapedes, McGraw-Hill.

Mervyn, L. (1986). Thorsons' complete guide to vitamins and minerals, Thorsons.

Scott, T. and Brewer, M. (1983). Concise encyclopedia of biochemistry, Walter de Gruyter.

Stenesh, J. (1975). Dictionary of biochemistry, John Wiley and Sons.

The encyclopedia of the biological sciences, (1983). Edited by P. Gray, Second Edition Van Nostrand.

Van Nostrand's scientific encyclopedia, (1983). Edited by D. M. Considine and G. D. Considine, Sixth Edition, Van Nostrand.

W. B. Saunders' atomic energy encyclopedia in the life sciences, (1964). Edited by C. Shilling, W. B. Saunders.

Yudkin, J. (1985). The penguin encyclopedia of nutrition, Penguin Books.

Textbooks

Bell, G. H., Davison, J. N. and Emslie-Smyth, D. (1972). Textbook of physiology and biochemistry, Eight Edition, Churchill Livingstone.

Bohinski, H. C. (1979). Modern concepts in biochemistry, Third Edition, Allyn and Bacon.

Bowman, C. and Rand, M. J. (1980). Textbook of pharmacology, Second Edition, Blackwell Scientific Publications.

Burton, B. T. (1976). Human nutrition, Third Edition, McGraw-Hill.

Davidson and Passmore's human nutrition and dietetics, (1986). 8th Edition, Edited by R. Passmore and M. A. Eastwood, Churchill Livingstone.

Ganong, F. (1987). Review of medical physiology, Thirteenth Edition, Lange Medical Publications.

Gibney, M. J. (1986). Nutrition, diet and health, Cambridge University Press.

Goodman and Gillman's the pharmacological basis of therapeutics, (1985). Seventh Edition, Edited by A. G. Gilman, L. S. Goodman, T. W. Rall and F. Murad, Macmillan.

Green, J. H. (1980). An introduction to human physiology, Fourth (SI) Revised Edition, Oxford University Press.

Gurr, M. I. (1984). Role of fats in food and nutrition, Elsevier Applied

Science Publishers.

Gurr, M. I. and James, A. T. (1975). Lipid biochemistry, Second Edition, Chapman and Hall.

Guyton, A. C. (2006). Textbook of medical physiology, Eleventh Edition, W. B. Saunders.

Katzung, B. G. (Editor) (1984). Basic clinical pharmacology, 2nd Edition, Lange Medical Publications.

Lehninger, A. L. (1982). Principles of Biochemistry, Worth Publishers Inc.

Lloyde, L. E., McDonald, B. E. and Crampton, E. W. (1978). Fundamentals of nutrition, Second Edition, W. H. Freeman and Co.

McDonald, P., Edwards, R. A. and Greenhalgh, J. F. D. (1988). Animal nutrition, Longman, Scientific and Technical.

Metzler, D. E. (1977). Biochemistry: the chemical reactions of living cells, Academic Press.

Murray, R. K., Granner, D. K., Mayes, P. A. and Rodwell, V. W. (1990). Harper's biochemistry, Twenty-second Edition, Lange Medical Books.

Ottaway, J. H. and Apps, D. K. (1984). Biochemistry, Fourth Edition, Baillière Tyndall.

Peterson, C. R. (1983). Essentials of human biochemistry, Pitman Books.

Smith, E. L., Hill, R. L., Lehman, I. R., Lefkowitz, R. J., Handler, P. and White, A. (1983). Principles of biochemistry: mammalian biochemistry, Seventh Edition McGraw-Hill.

Taylor, T. G. (1978). Principles of human nutrition, The Institute of Biology Series No 94, Edward Arnold.

Vander, A. J., Sherman, J. H. and Luciane, D. S. (1984). Human physiology: the mechanism of body function, Fourth Edition, McGraw-Hill.

Wills, E. D. (1985). Biochemical basis of medicine, John Wright and Sons.

Reference Works

Assmann, G. (1982). Lipid metabolism and atherosclerosis, F. K. Schattauer Verlag.

Bender, A. E. and Bender, D. A. (1986). Food tables, Oxford University Press.

Biochemical nomenclature and related documents, (1978). International Union of Biochemistry, as reprinted for the Biochemical Society by Spottiswoode Ballantyne Press.

Biological handbooks (new series) Vol II: Human health and disease, (1977). Edited by P. L. Altman and D. Dittmer Katz, Fed. Amer. Soc. Exp. Biol., Bethesda, Maryland.

Biological handbooks: blood and other body fluids (1961). Edited by P. L. Altman and D. S. Dittmer, Fed. Amer. Soc. Exp. Biol., Bethesda, Maryland.

Biological handbooks: metabolism, (1968). Edited by P. L. Altman and D. S. Dittmer, Fed. Amer. Soc. Exp. Biol., Bethesda, Maryland.

CRC handbook of biochemistry: selected data for molecular biology, (1970). 2nd Edition, Edited by H. A. Sober, CRC Press.

CRC handbook of chemistry and physics, (1981). 62nd Edition, Edited by R. C. Weast and M. J. Astle, CRC Press.

CRC handbook of eicosanoids: prostaglandins and related lipids, Vol I (Part A): Biochemical aspects (1987). Edited by A. L. Willis, CRC Press.

CRC handbook series. Nutrition and food: Section E, nutritional disorders, Vol I. Effects of nutrient excesses and toxicities in animals and man, (1977). Edited by M. Rechcigl, Jr., CRC Press.

Food and agriculture organisation: energy yielding components of food and computation of caloric values. (1947). F.A.O. Nutrition Division.

Food, nutrition and climate (1982). Edited by K. Blaxter and L. Fowden, Applied Science Publishers.

Geigy Scientific Tables: Eight revised and enlarged edition, Edited by C. Lentner, Ciba-Geigy.

Handbook of vitamins: nutritional, biochemical and clinical aspects (1984). Edited by L. J. Machlin, Marcel Dekker.

Nutrient interactions, (1988). Edited by C. E. Bodwell and J. W. Erdman, Jr., Marcel Dekker.

Osborne, D. R. and Voogt, P. (1978). The analysis of nutrients in foods, Academic Press.

Paul, A. A. and Southgate, D. A. T. (1978). McCance and Widdowson's the composition of foods, Fourth Edition, H. M. Stationary Office London.

Paul, A. A., Southgate, D. A. T., and Russell, J. (1980). First supplement to McCance and Widdowson's the composition of foods, H. M. Stationary Office London.

Reeds, P. J., (2000). "Dispensable and indispensable amino acids for humans", *American Society for Nutritional Sciences, Supplement.* 1835S–1840S.

Recommended dietary allowances (1989). Tenth Edition, Food and Nutrition Board, National Academy of Sciences - National Research Council, US.

Requirements of vitamin A, iron, folate and vitamin B12 (1988). Report of joint FAO/WHO expert consultation. Food and Agriculture Organisation of the United Nations, Rome.

Shamberger, R. J. (1983). Biochemistry of the elements: Vol 2. Biochemistry of selenium, Plenum Press.

Trace elements in human and animal nutrition: Vol 2 (1986). Fifth Edition, Edited by W. Mertz, Orlando, Academic Press.

Van Dorp, P. A. (1973). Essential fatty acids and prostaglandins: Vol 2. Butterworths.

World Health Organisation: handbook on human nutritional requirements (1974). Monograph Series No. 61, WHO in collaboration with the Food and Agriculture Organisation of the United Nations.

Web Sources

Dietary Reference Intakes, (1997 – 2011). National Academies Press.

Dietary Reference Intakes for Calcium, Phosphorous, Magnesium, Vitamin D, and Fluoride (1997);

Dietary Reference Intakes for Thiamin, Riboflavin, Niacin, Vitamin B6, Folate, Vitamin B12, Pantothenic Acid, Biotin, and Choline (1998);

Dietary Reference Intakes for Vitamin C, Vitamin E, Selenium, and Carotenoids (2000);

Dietary Reference Intakes for Vitamin A, Vitamin K, Arsenic, Boron, Chromium, Copper, Iodine, Iron, Manganese, Molybdenum, Nickel, Silicon, Vanadium, and Zinc (2001);

Dietary Reference Intakes for Energy, Carbohydrate, Fiber, Fat, Fatty Acids, Cholesterol, Protein, and Amino Acids (2002/2005);

Dietary Reference Intakes for Calcium and Vitamin D (2011);

Note: These reports may be accessed via: *www.nap.edu* .

Dietary Reference Intakes (DRIs): Estimated Average Requirements. Food and Nutrition Board, Institute of Medicine, National Academies. Life Stage. Group.
https://fnic.nal.usda.gov/sites/fnic.nal.usda.gov/files/uploads/recommended_ intakes_individuals.pdf [modified: 16 December 2015].

United States Department of Agriculture, National Agricultural Library (USDA, NAL), DRI Tables and Application Reports,
https://fnic.nal.usda.gov/dietary-guidance/dietary-reference-intakes [modified: 30 April 2016].
https://fnic.nal.usda.gov/dietary-guidance/dietary-reference-intakes/ dri-tables-and-application-reports [retrieved: 28 September 2016].

Dietary Reference Intakes (DRIs) are developed and published by the Institute of Medicine (IOM). The DRIs represent the most current scientific knowledge on nutrient needs of healthy populations.

Dietary Reference Intakes for Energy, Carbohydrate, Fiber, Fat, Fatty Acids, Cholesterol, Protein, and Amino Acids (Macronutrients), (2005). National Academies Press. *http://www.nap.edu/catalog/10490/ dietary-reference-intakes-for-energy-carbohydrate-fiber-fat-fatty-acids-cholesterol-protein-and-amino-acids-macronutrients* [modified: 7 April

2016].

Linus Pauling Institute, Micronutrient Information Center. Oregon State University. Choline, *http://lpi.oregonstate.edu/mic/other-nutrients/choline* [retrieved: 29 April 2016].

Linus Pauling Institute, Micronutrient Information Center. Oregon State University. Essential Fatty Acids, *http://lpi.oregonstate.edu/mic/other-nutrients/essential-fatty-acids* [retrieved: 28 September 2016].

The Linus Pauling Institute is a valuable authoritative source of information on the nutrients.

Payne, P.R., (1971). Reference protein patterns, 1–8, *ftp://ftp.fao.org/docrep/fao/meeting/009/ae906e/ae906e25.pdf* [modified: 12 October 2016].

Supplements-And-Health.com. (2016). Lesser Known Facts About Tryptophan Side Effects. *http://www.supplements-and-health.com/tryptophan-side-effects.html* [retrieved: 21 October 2016].

University of Maryland Medical Centre. (2016). Phenylalanine, *http://umm.edu/health/medical/altmed/supplement/phenylalanine* [retrieved: 17 October 2016].

US Department of Agriculture, National Agricultural Library. (2016). DRI Nutrient Reports. https://fnic.nal.usda.gov/dietary-guidance/dietary-reference-intakes/dri-nutrient-reports [retrieved, 18 October 2016].

Wikipedia. (2016). "Essential amino acid", *https://en.wikipedia.org/wiki/Essential_amino_acid* [modified: 11 October 2016].

About the Author

Richard Rydon

Richard Rydon is an award-winning science fiction novelist. His three books in the Luper Series, The Oortian Summer (2007), The Omega Wave (2008) and The Palomar Paradox: A SETI Mystery (2011), have been given excellent reviews.

Richard's second novel, The Omega Wave, was selected as one of the finalists in the Science Fiction Category of the Reader Views Literary Awards and was awarded an Honorary Mention (Third Place) in the Reviewers Choice Awards in 2009.

His third novel, The Palomar Paradox, won the Bronze/3rd Place award in the Romance Category of the Feathered Quill Book Awards in 2014.

Richard is an honours science graduate. He has also obtained numerous certificates and diplomas in Psychology, Counselling, Theology, and a Diplôme de Cuisine Française. He is a prolific writer and has published over 300 papers, articles and poems, in scientific journals, magazines and local papers to date.

He has also published a second edition of his anthology of poetry, titled A Golden Fuchsia-Laden Girl (2011), containing 100 poems.

About the Science Fiction Novels in the Luper Series

The Oortian Summer

'The Oortian Summer' is a romantic science fiction adventure involving co-worker relationships in an astronomical observatory as two massive comets approach the Earth. The unusual twist in the story involves a perilous attempt, proposed by Luper, the lead character, to bring the comets even closer to Earth to prevent a catastrophic geomagnetic flip.

The Omega Wave

'The Omega Wave' is a gothic science fiction novel. Aided and abetted by Quade their boss, Luper and Frieda progress secretly and meticulously, to develop biological computers called neurospheres. Working in the shadow of a rogue American Embassy, they first conceal but later reveal what they have seen and done.

The Palomar Paradox: A SETI Mystery

'The Palomar Paradox' sees Luper back in an astronomical observatory searching for signs of extraterrestrial intelligence. He finds himself working with Leila, a young girl recovering from leukaemia, and Karina, an experienced astronomer, among others. As their research continues, unusual signals are picked up by their radio telescope. The signals are explained, one by one, until … !

About Richard Rydon's Poetry

A Golden Fuchsia-Laden Girl

'A Golden Fuchsia-Laden Girl' is an anthology of one hundred poems of whimsy, innocence and longing, by Richard Rydon, written and revised between 1957 and 2011. Twenty poems have been added in this second edition.

About Richard Rydon's Non-Fiction Books

Matter, Energy and Mentality: Exploring Metaphysical Reality

His non-fiction book, 'Matter, Energy and Mentality: Exploring Metaphysical Reality', was published in 2012. 'Matter, Energy and Mentality' is a book of speculative non-fiction. It covers the relationships between Matter, Energy and Mentality, using Energy Redistribution (Unnecessary Action) as a common feature in the Universe.

Profiles of the Nutrients

'Profiles of the Nutrients — 1. Carbohydrate, Lipid, and Protein' published in 2016, is the first book in a series about the nutrients which are essential for human life.

The other books in the series will be titled as follows:

'Profiles of the Nutrients — 2. Minerals and Trace Elements'.
'Profiles of the Nutrients — 3. Water-Soluble and Fat-Soluble
Vitamins